BrainChip
for
Microbiology

USMLE Step 1 Review

BrainChip
for
Microbiology

Scott Lee

MD-MPH candidate

Howard Hughes Medical Institute
Fellow 1999-2000

Harvard University School
of Public Health

UCLA School of Medicine

**Blackwell
Science**

© 2001 by Blackwell Science, Inc.

Blackwell Science, Inc.

EDITORIAL OFFICES:
Commerce Place, 350 Main Street, Malden, Massachusetts 02148, USA
Osney Mead, Oxford OX2 0EL, England
25 John Street, London WC1N 2BL, England
23 Ainslie Place, Edinburgh EH3 6AJ, Scotland
54 University Street, Carlton, Victoria 3053, Australia
OTHER EDITORIAL OFFICES:
Blackwell Wissenschafts-Verlag GmbH, Kurfürstendamm 57, 10707 Berlin, Germany
Blackwell Science KK, MG Kodenmacho Building, 7-10 Kodenmacho Nihombashi,
   Chuo-ku, Tokyo 104, Japan
Iowa State University Press, A Blackwell Science Company, 2121 S. State Avenue, Ames,
   Iowa 50014-8300, USA

DISTRIBUTORS:
USA
   Blackwell Science, Inc.
   Commerce Place
   350 Main Street
   Malden, Massachusetts 02148
   Telephone orders: (800) 215-1000
      or (781) 388-8250;
   Fax orders: (781) 388-8270
Canada
   Login Brothers Book Company
   324 Saulteaux Crescent
   Winnipeg, Manitoba R3J 3T2
   Telephone orders: (204) 837-2987

Australia
   Blackwell Science Pty, Ltd.
   54 University Street
   Carlton, Victoria 3053
   Telephone orders: 03-9347-0300
   Fax orders: 03-9349-3016
Outside North America and Australia
   Blackwell Science, Ltd.
   c/o Marston Book Services, Ltd.
   P.O. Box 269
   Abingdon
   Oxon OX14 4YN
   England
   Telephone orders: 44-01235-465500
   Fax orders: 44-01235-465555

Acquisitions: Beverly Copland
Development: Julia Casson
Production: GraphCom Corporation
Marketing Manager: Toni Fournier
Printed and bound by Western Press

Printed in the United States of America
01 02 03 04 5 4 3 2 1

The Blackwell Science logo is a trade mark of Blackwell Science Ltd., registered at the United Kingdom Trade Marks Registry

Library of Congress Cataloging-in-Publication Data

Lee, Scott, 1974-
   Brain chip for microbiology / by Scott Lee.
      p. ; cm.
   ISBN 0-632-04568-X
   1. Microbiology—Outlines, syllabi, etc. 2. Medical microbiology—Outlines, syllabi, etc.
I. Title.
   [DNLM: I. Microbiology. QW 4 L481b 2001]
   QR62 .L44 2001
   615'.01—dc21

00-067485

DEDICATION

This book is dedicated to the missionary physicians of Hospital Vozandes HCJB in the Amazon jungle, and their tireless efforts and labor of eternal value, to ameliorate suffering and serve the marginalized and destitute who do not have access to health care.

Figure Credits

The following figures were borrowed with permission from:

Bannister, Barbara A: Figures 1.2, 3.2, 3.3, 4.2, 4.3, 8.1, 8.2, 8.4, 8.8, 9.1, 9.2, 9.3, 10.5, 10.6, 10.7, 11.1, 11.2, 11.3, 12.1, 12.2, 12.4, 13.1, 14.1, 15.1, 15.2, 16.4, 17.1, 22.1, 23.2, 23.3, 23.4, 25.2, 26.2, 26.3, 26.4, 27.1, 27.2, 27.3 (Figures 2.4a,b, 2.5, 2.8, 3.1, 3.2, 3.6, 3.8, 5.21, 5.24, 5.27, 6.8, 6.12, 6.13, 7.4a,b, 7.7, 7.10, 8.3, 8.11, 8.15, 8.16a,b,d, 8.18, 9.2, 9.8, 9.9, 9.13b, 11.2, 11.10, 13.13, 13.14b, 15.3, 20.5, 24.6, 24.10b, 24.13a, 25.1, and 79.1 in *Infectious Diseases* © 2000 Blackwell Science, Ltd.)

Crissey, John Thorne: Figures 19.1, 19.3, 19.6, 19.7, 19.8, 19.9, 20.7, 21.1, 21.2,21.3, 21.4 (Figures 4.7, 4.12, 4.14, 5.6, 5.8, 5.14, 5.27, 5.37, 7.1, 7.5, and 7.13 in *Manual of Medical Mycology* © 1995 Blackwell Science, Ltd.

Elliot, TSJ: Figures 1.1, 8.3, 8.5, 8.6, 8.7, 9.4, 10.1, 19.2 (Plates 2, 4, 11, 13, 14, 25, 29, 59 in *Lecture Notes on Medical Microbiology* © 1997 Blackwell Science, Ltd.)

Gillespie, Stephen: Figure 24.2 (Diagram on page 52 borrowed in *Medical Microbiology at a Glance* © 2000 Blackwell Science, Ltd.)

Graham-Brown, Robin AC: Figures 10.2, 12.3, 20.2, 20.3, 20.4, 20.5 (Figures 3.2, 3.11, 4.1, 4.2, 4.6, and 4.7 in *Lecture Notes on Dermatology* © 1996 Blackwell Science, Ltd.

Holton, John: Figures 4.1, 7.4, 11.4, 11.5, 19.4, 20.1, 22.2, 22.4, 24.1, 26.5, 26.6 (Figures 3.1, 7.3, 13.1, 20.2, 25.1, 40.1, 45.1, 74.2, 75.2, 78.1, 80.1, and 80.2 in *Problems in Medical Microbiology* © 1995 Blackwell Science, Ltd.)

Hunter, John A: Figure 19.5 (Figure 15.45 in *Clinical Dermatology* © 1992 Blackwell Science, Ltd.)

Smalligan, Roger, MD: Figures 3.1, 7.1, 7.2, 7.3, 7.5, 10.3, 10.4, 14.2, 16.1, 16.2, 16.3, 20.6, 22.3, 23.1, 25.1, 26.1, 26.7

NOTE: Figures in parenthesis indicate figure numbers in the borrowed source.

TABLE OF CONTENTS

FOREWORD

It is a pleasure to introduce this important book by a recent graduate of the Harvard School of Public Health. Scott Lee has written an excellent introductory book on microbiology that presents key concepts through clinical vignettes and photographs. Many of the photographs come from Scott's clinical experiences during field placements in Thailand, Ecuador, the Philippines, and El Salvador. *BrainChip for Microbiology* is designed to prepare students for the microbiology component of the Step 1 medical qualifying examination, and it will also be of value to clinicians seeking a broad review of microbiology and for students in fields such as public health who seek an introduction to infectious diseases.

The author is a talented young health professional who has completed 3 years of clinical training at UCLA, a year as a Howard Hughes Fellow at the National Institutes of Health, and a year earning the MPH degree at the Harvard School of Public Health. *BrainChip for Microbiology* is enhanced by his laboratory experiences, his extensive international experience, and his year of studies in public health. This book is an excellent start to a new series for medical students and health professionals. It will be a valuable resource for its readers.

James H. Ware, PhD
Academic Dean of the Harvard School of Public Health

PREFACE

BrainChip for Microbiology was written out of the need for a complete review book in microbiology, one which we could not find while studying for boards. There are three major components to such a book. A concise, succinct, and high-yield text that is complete—in and of itself—for USMLE Step 1 is a given in any review text. Such a text would not only cover the basic science of microbiology with all its mechanistic details, pathways, and biochemical details, but it would also include the clinical presentations of infectious disease. Further, photographs make up a significant portion of Step 1—of both microscopy and cultures and patient pictures. We have attempted to address all these issues in this text.

With the understanding that the student has had a standard microbiology course, *BrainChip for Microbiology* is written for rapid review of microbiology in 4 to 7 days with the most essential information provided. It is intended to be used in conjunction with a more comprehensive text if used for a course. With sufficient background, however, it can be read alone.

BrainChip for Microbiology is organized by microorganism groups. In each section is a "History of the present illness," as it is often presented on the examination. Only the most salient facts are included, which is often a very brief HPI. This may not be indicative of many boards questions in which extraneous material is often present. You may want to practice thinking about a differential diagnosis and etiologic organism by only reading the HPI and guessing the bug. You will find that many of the organisms have similar presentation and therefore have similar HPIs. However, where there are subtle differences, these are in bold type.

After the organism name is given, its disease, and its microbiologic and biochemical mechanisms of pathogenesis are given. We have included what we believe is sufficient for Step 1, but examiners have a way of asking the most obscure facts. We advise that you use this text in conjunction with your class microbiology notes if you desire more detail on any subject.

Basic diagnosis mechanisms and treatment are also outlined. These have been updated in correlation with CDC guidelines for 2001. Often diagnoses will be clinical judgments, rather than specific tests. It would be prudent in such cases to note the differences in clinical presentation with similar organisms.

Finally, "classic" pictures are presented where relevant. Memorize these pictures! They will likely appear in one form or another when a JPEG appears on your screen during Step 1.

BrainChip for Microbiology has been prepared with a great deal of research and corroboration with multiple authorities. However, as with any text, there are bound to be shortcomings. We welcome and encourage your suggestions, advice, and vitriolic attacks.

It is our hope that you find this text beneficial and an efficient use of your time. We sincerely wish you success on Step 1 and your exams.

ACKNOWLEDGMENTS

I am indebted to many individuals for the publication of this work.

I would like to thank Julia Casson, Bill Deluise, and Beverly Copland at Blackwell Science for all of their support and kindness. The publication of this text would not have been possible without their hard work and the efforts they put forth.

I would like to thank the Howard Hughes Medical Institute, James Gavin III, Director; Donald Harter, Director Emeritus; and Barbara Ziff, Administrative Director, for their support during the tenure of which this book was written.

I would like to thank Ugonna Iroku, Marcus Ko, and Deidre Larrier, Harvard Medical School, for their critical reading of the manuscript.

I am indebted to Roger Smalligan for his mentorship in Ecuador and the numerous pictures in this text. The amazing pathology and clinical presentations of the patients of the Pastaza region of the Amazon jungle would not have been documented in this book without his efforts.

Finally, I am indebted to my parents, Dongha and Kyung Lee, and to my brother, Grant, for their love and devotion for a quarter century.

—Scott Lee

ABBREVIATIONS

ABX	Antibiotics
ADP	Adenosine diphosphate
AIDS	Acquired immunodeficiency syndrome
ATP	Adenosine triphosphate
BBB	Blood-brain barrier
BSE	Bovine spongioencephalitis
BUN	Blood urea nitrogen
CMV	Cytomegalovirus
CNS	Central nervous system
CPE	Cytopathogenic effect
CR	Creatinine
CSF	Cerebrospinal fluid
CXR	Chest x-ray
CT	Computed tomography
DIC	Disseminated intravascular coagulation
DNA	Deoxyribonucleic acid
DTH	Delayed-type hypersensitivity
EBV	Epstein-Barr virus
EEE	Eastern equine encephalitis
EMB	Eosin methylene blue
FTA-ABs	Fluorescent treponemal antibody-absorption test
GI	gastrointestinal
GM+	Gram positive
H2S	Hydrogen sulfide gas
HCT	Hematocrit
HIV	Human immunodeficiency virus
HPV	Human papillomavirus
HSV I	Herpes simplex virus type I
HUS	Hemolytic uremic syndrome
IUGR	Intrauterine growth restriction
LAT	Latency-associated transcript
LFT	Liver function tests
LPS	Lipopolysaccharide
MMR	Measles-mumps-rubella
MRSA	Methicillin resistant *S. aureus*
OLM	Ocular larva migrans
PE	Physical examination
PCP	Pneumocystis pneumonia

PCR	Polymerase chain reaction
PHN	Postherpetic neuralgia
PID	Pelvic inflammatory disease
PMN	Polymorphonuclear
PT	Patient
RBC	Red blood cell
RES	Reticuloendothelial system
RLL	Right lower lobe
RLQ	Right lower quadrant
RNA	Ribonucleic acid
rRNA	Ribosomal RNA
RSV	Respiratory syncytial virus
RUQ	Right upper quadrant
SSPE	Subacute schlerosing panecencephalitis
SX	Symptoms
TCA	Trichloroacetic
TB	Tuberculosis
TX	Treatment
UG	Urogenitary
VLM	Visceral larva migrans
VSG	Varient science glycoprotein
WBC	White blood cell
WHO	World Health Organization
YO	Year old

BACTERIA

CHAPTER 1: OBLIGATE INTRACELLULAR ORGANISMS

History of present illness: 25 yo sexually active woman reports bilateral lower abdominal pain for 4 weeks with varying intensity. She has had no diarrhea, vomiting, or dysuria. On PE, she exhibits severe cervical motion tenderness. Clear discharge is noted from an obtained cervical specimen. The patient refuses treatment but subsequently returns to clinic with spiking fevers to 39° C, peritoneal signs, and significant right upper quadrant pain. Ultrasound examination shows an enlarged liver with fluid collection and tuboovarian mass. Most likely etiological agent:

Chlamydia trachomatis: PID with Fitz-Hugh–Curtis perihepatitis (Figure 1.1)
Disease: Types ABC Conjunctivitis → bacterial superinfection → corneal scarring → blindness
   Types DEFGK: Genital tract infections: nongonococcal (although clinically similar) urethritis in men; PID, tuboovarian abscess in women → infertility, perihepatitis **(Fitz-Hugh–Curtis syndrome)**, neonatal conjunctivitis
   Types L1-L3: Lymphogranuloma venereum, very **tender** lesions on genitals
Characteristics and pathogenesis: Obligate intracellular parasites require host ATP. Transmitted in humans via sexual, birth canal, or finger or eye contact only. Life cycle: **Elementary body** enters human cells → changes into metabolically active **reticulate body** → reproduces as **daughter** elementary bodies
Diagnosis: Antigen testing in STD cases; Giemsa stain of conjunctival scrapings
Treatment: doxycycline and ceftriaxone. Always treat as though patient has gonorrhea. Concomitant infection is high.

BACTERIA

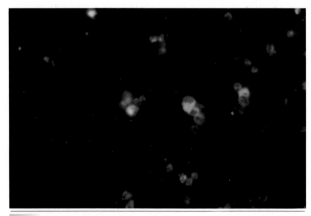

FIGURE 1.1 *Chlamydia trachomatis.*

OBLIGATE INTRACELLULAR ORGANISMS—cont'd

History of present illness: 39 yo zoo worker, who specializes in Far Eastern birds, develops a hacking cough 3 weeks previously. The cough is nonproductive and without hemoptysis. PE is unremarkable, and lungs are apparently clear. CXR shows diffuse infiltrates without specific lobar involvement. Most likely etiological agent:

Chylamydia psittaci
Disease: Atypical pneumonia
Characteristics and pathogenesis: Obligate intracellular parasites are transmitted via inhalation of bacteria, especially those individuals with a predilection for smelling bird droppings.
Diagnosis: Clinical, CXR
Treatment: erythromycin

♦   ♦   ♦

History of present illness: 27 yo woman from **Idaho** moves into a **dog-breeding** station. There, she notices small welts on her lower extremities but remains unconcerned. After 3 days, she presents to a dermatology clinic with a rash on her hands and feet, and she is treated with corticosteroids. Subsequently, the patient returns to clinic; the maculopapular rash has spread to her trunks, and numerous petechiae are present. In addition, she has fevers to 38.7° C and a generalized headache. A CBC shows a rise in the BUN. Most likely etiological agent:

Rickettsia rickettsii
Disease: Rocky Mountain spotted fever; **centripetal** maculopapular rash (inward from extremities to trunk), fever, and headache
Characteristics and pathogenesis: Obligate intracellular organisms transmitted by dog tick; reproduce by **binary fission**
Diagnosis: Weil-Felix test: positive
Treatment: tetracycline

History of present illness: 39 yo man develops influenza-like symptoms of malaise and weakness for 1 day. The patient has developed a severe headache that is getting progressively worse. A maculopapular rash erupts on his trunk and axillary folds and has begun to spread peripherally. The patient seems unable to concentrate and loses consciousness. Numerous persons in his village have had the same symptoms. Note: There is no rash on his feet, palms, or face. Most likely etiological agent:

Rickettsia prowazekii
Disease: Epidemic typhus: development of meningoencephalitis; **centrifugal** rash (outward from trunk to extremities)
Characteristics and pathogenesis: Transmitted human to **human** by human body louse in Asia and Africa. Human needed in life cycle **versus** *Rickettsia rickettsii*
Diagnosis: Weil-Felix test: positive
Treatment: tetracycline

♦   ♦   ♦

History of present illness: 52 yo woman reports mild headache, myalgias, and fever to 39° C. Similar rash to the one observed in the previous patient is noted, but it appears to be localized only to the trunk and has not spread in the last 2 days. No one in the village has had similar symptoms. Most likely etiological agent:

Rickettsia typhi
Disease: Endemic typhus
Characteristics and pathogenesis: Transmitted by fleas in unclean areas
Diagnosis: Weil-Felix test: positive
Treatment: tetracycline

BACTERIA

Obligate Intracellular Organisms—cont'd

History of present illness: 26 yo sheep rancher presents with fever for the previous 2 days, malaise, headache, and generalized influenza-like symptoms, which is the initial diagnosis. He returns 2 days later with increased cough without sputum production. There is no rash. PE shows a tender right upper quadrant. CXR shows diffuse infiltrates. Blood work shows an increased white blood cell count and elevated LFTs. The following organism is revealed:

Coxiella burnetti

Disease: Q fever: influenza-like symptoms; advances to an atypical pneumonia, hepatitis. **No** rash

Characteristics and pathogenesis: Transmitted by aerosol of cattle and sheep products (Figure 1.2)

Diagnosis: Weil-Felix test: **negative**

Treatment: tetracycline

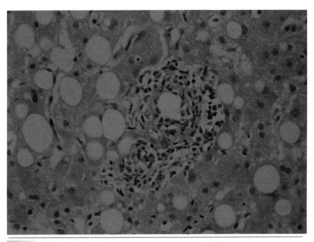

Figure 1.2   *Coxiella burnetti.*

CHAPTER 2: ORGANISMS WITH NO CELL WALL

History of present illness: 18 yo pre-med female university student complains of cough that has lasted 4 weeks without sputum production and without hemoptysis, generalized mild malaise, and weakness. CXR shows a lower lobe bronchial pneumonia. Patient is otherwise without complaint and desires to get back to class as soon as possible. Most likely etiological agent:

Mycoplasma pneumoniae
Disease: Atypical "walking" pneumonia, the patient feels generally well, CXR looks **"horrible."**
Characteristics and pathogenesis: No cell wall therefore resists **penicillins** and cannot be gram-stained tested. **Cholesterol** in cell membrane, **"egg yoke"** morphology is observed on **Eaton's agar.** Acts by inducing epithelial cell death and stopping cilliary motion. Anti-RBC autoantibodies **(cold agglutinins)** produced by cross-rxn.
Diagnosis: Clinical by history and x-ray, increased cold agglutinins, if necessary
Treatment: erythromycin, azithromycin

♦   ♦   ♦

History of present illness: 54 yo sexually active man complains of difficulty urinating and dysuria. He has had mild fever for 1 week, and on PE, the patient has a small penile discharge. Rectal examination reveals a boggy and tender prostate. Urine is sent for culture after the prostate examination, which reveals the following organism:

Ureaplasma urealyticum
Disease: Nongonococcal urethritis, **progresses to prostatitis,** epididymitis, chorioamnionitis
Characteristics and pathogenesis: No cell wall; urease is positive
Diagnosis: Clinical
Treatment: tetracycline or doxycycline

BACTERIA

CHAPTER 3: GRAM-NEGATIVE RODS (GI)

History of present illness: 32 yo traveler returns from Southeast Asia. She presents with abdominal cramps, nonbilious vomiting without blood, and profuse diarrhea. She has a very dry mouth, eyes with little lacrimation, and no apparent sweat on other parts of her body. Stools appear as "rice water" and are without blood as well. Blood pressure is 90/60, and the patient is unable to maintain concentration. Most likely etiological agent:

Vibrio cholera
Disease: Cholera. Massive watery **rice-water** diarrhea, fecal-oral transmission

Characteristics and pathogenesis: Comma-shaped, single flagellum; **mucinase** to colonize intestine, **bipartite enterotoxin:** (1) **B** subunit binds **GM1 gangliosides** on enterocytes; (2) **A** subunit activates **adenylate cyclase via ADP ribosylation of G protein** → ↑ **cAMP** → ↑ **secretion** and ↓ **absorption of Na + Cl** → **secretory diarrhea**

Diagnosis: Clinical

Treatment: Supportive, oral rehydration solution; WHO solution

♦   ♦   ♦

History of present illness: 32 yo patient presents with diarrhea of 2-day duration. Stool was initially watery and clear, but it is now bloody. The patient has abdominal pain, malaise, and fever to 39° C. Culture of stool reveals the following organism:

Campylobacter jejuni and intestinalis
Disease: Enterocolitis; diarrhea, often bloody

Characteristics and pathogenesis: Comma or S-shaped, enterotoxin pathogenesis, urease negative

Diagnosis: Blood agar with antibiotics; *C. jejuni* grows at **42° C,** nalidixic acid–**sensitive, oxidase positive;** *C. intestinalis* grows at **25° C,** nalidixic acid–**resistant, oxidase negative**

Treatment: ciprofloxacin

GRAM-NEGATIVE RODS (GI)—cont'd

History of present illness: 54 yo male presents with epigastric abdominal pain. He has had no vomitus or diarrhea. The pain is associated with food. Upper GI endoscopy reveals multiple gastric lesions and ulcers. A course of antibiotic therapy along with a proton pump inhibitor alleviates the patient's symptoms. A blood test for the following organism would be positive for:

H. pylori
Disease: Peptic ulcer disease, gastritis
Characteristics and pathogenesis: Urease positive, NH_3 production, protected against acidic stomach environment
Diagnosis: Blood test for *H. pylori* titer, stomach ulcer biopsy (indicated to assess for cancer)
Treatment: Triple therapy: Antacid (Proton pump inhibitor, H_2 blocker, or Bismuth sulfate) tetracycline, metronidazole

◆   ◆   ◆

History of present illness: 14 yo returns from an **egg salad** picnic **6 hrs** ago and symptoms of vomiting, diarrhea, fever, and abdominal pains ensue. The symptoms continue for 4 days and the patient does not seek medical care. All symptoms resolve on their own, and the patient returns to school. Most likely etiological agent:

Salmonella enteritidis
Disease: Gastroenteritis via cholera-like toxin. **Large inoculum** required because organism is **peptic acid susceptible**
Characteristics and pathogenesis: K antigen/Vi antigen **flagella antigenic variation, motile**
Diagnosis: Does **NOT** ferment **lactose;** produces H_2S gas
Treatment: ceftriaxone, ciprofloxacin, supportive treatment, no Imodium

GRAM-NEGATIVE RODS (GI)—cont'd

History of present illness: 32 yo man travels to Ecuador. Within
3 weeks, he develops gradual onset of fever and abdominal pain.
Hepatosplenomegaly is noted. Patient refuses treatment; intestinal
perforation with peritonitis ensues within 1 week; emergent surgery
is required. A characteristic rash is noted (Figure 3.1). Most likely
etiological agent:

Salmonella typhi

Disease: Typhoid fever. Fever, RLQ abdominal pain from hepatic, gallbladder involvement; rose spots on abdomen

Characteristics and pathogenesis: K antigen and Vi antigen **flagella
antigenic variation**

Diagnosis: Does **NOT** ferment **lactose;** produces H_2S gas; **motile**

Treatment: ceftriaxone, ciprofloxacin

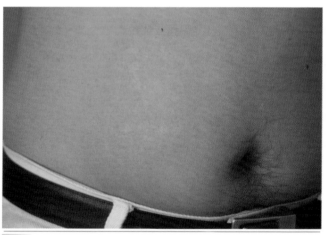

FIGURE 3.1 Rose spots. © Dr. Roger Smalligan.

GRAM-NEGATIVE RODS (GI)—cont'd

History of present illness: 35 yo man presents with diarrhea of 1 week duration; characterized by blood and mucus. Fever to 40° C and abdominal pain are concurrent with other symptoms. The patient does not vomit. His symptoms resolve with prompt antimicrobial treatment. Most likely etiological agent:

Shigella
Disease: Dysentery by *S. dysentariae, S. sonnei, S. flexneri, S. boydii*
Characteristics and pathogenesis: Small innoculum < 1000 organisms required; transmitted by feces fingers, flies, food, (fecal-oral); **nonmotile** colonic mucosal **invasion** and cell death → bloody stool; does **NOT** enter bloodstream versus *Salmonella*
Diagnosis: No H₂S gas; nonlactose fermenting on EMB; MacConkey's agar; **PMNs** in stool
Treatment: ciprofloxacin, no antimotility agents

♦   ♦   ♦

History of present illness: 32 yo woman presents with dysuria and suprapubic pain of 3 days duration. She is treated for a urinary tract infection. Patient returns 2 weeks later in greater pain, dysuria, and patient is febrile to 39.5° C. Patient admits that she was not compliant with the treatment regimen. On PE, patient is tender bilaterally in the costovertebral angles. UA shows blood and pyuria. Most likely etiological agent:

Extraintestinal *Escherichia coli*

GRAM-NEGATIVE RODS (GI)—cont'd

History of present illness: 22 yo man traveling in Africa develops bloody diarrhea of 2 days duration. After having received no treatment and becoming severely dehydrated, the patient becomes neurologically impaired 1 week later. He is unable to communicate coherently and maintain consciousness. He has not urinated in 3 days. Stool sample is positive for fecal leukocytes. CBC reveals an Hct of 25, and the chem 7 reveals a BUN of 60. Most likely etiological agent:

Enteric *Escherichia coli:* HUS syndrome (Figure 3.2)
Disease: Enterocolitis, urinary tract infection, sepsis, neonatal meningitis
Characteristics and pathogenesis:
  Enterotoxigenic strains: **Heat labile** enterotoxin binds **GM1 ganglioside** receptor, activates adenylate cyclase via ADP ribosylation of G protein (as in cholera); results in **watery diarrhea**
  Enterohemorrhagic strains: **Verotoxin** inhibits 60s ribosome (as in Shigella) results in **bloody diarrhea; 0157:H7 type** causes **hemolytic-uremic syndrome** (triad of anemia, thrombocytopenia, renal failure) associated with fast-food outbreaks
  Enteroinvasive strains: Factor-mediated invasion of epithelial cells, sepsis; **bloody diarrhea with WBCs;** invasion mediated by endotoxin, enterotoxin, pilus, and capsule; capsular serotype via **O,H,K antigens**
Diagnosis: Clinical diagnosis; **ferments lactose** unlike other enterocolitic bugs (Figure 3.3)
Treatment: ceftriaxone

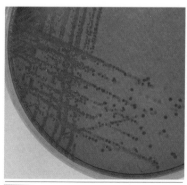

FIGURE 3.2 *Enteric Escherichia coli.*

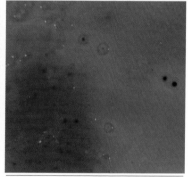

FIGURE 3.3 *Enteric Escherichia coli* at higher magnification.

CHAPTER 4: GRAM-NEGATIVE RODS (RESPIRATORY)

History of present illness: 3 yo child presents with fever to 39° C, headache, and photophobia. PE demonstrates tachycardia, clear lungs to auscultation, and mild nuchal rigidity. The child is irritable and crying. Most likely etiological agent:

Haemophilus influenzae (Figure 4.1)
Disease: *H. influenzae* meningitis, URI, pneumonia, sepsis
Characteristics and pathogenesis: Transmitted by respiratory droplets → oropharynx → nonencapsulated organism → otitis media, pneumonia; if **capsulated (type b polysaccharide capsule)** → bacteremia, meningitis, arthritis
Diagnosis: Gram stain, serotyping, **chocolate agar with NAD + heme** (factors: V, five and X, ten) for culture
Treatment: hospitalization, chloramphenicol, ceftriaxone

BACTERIA

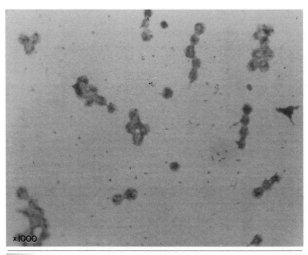
x1000

FIGURE 4.1 *Haemophilus influenzae.*

GRAM-NEGATIVE RODS (RESPIRATORY)—cont'd

History of present illness: 5 yo unvaccinated child presents with forceful spasmodic coughing of 2 week duration. Symptoms began with a mild cold 10 days previously, and symptoms have progressively worsened. Cough is followed by a high-pitched "oop" on inspiration and vomiting with copious mucus. PE reveals a left otitis media; x-ray exam shows a right lower lobe pneumonia. Most likely etiological agent:

Bordetella pertussis (Figure 4.2)

Disease: Whooping cough: paroxysmal hacking cough for 1 to 4 weeks; acute tracheobronchitis with URI symptoms; copious mucus; seizures, apnea, mental retardation, and paralysis are also associated; transmitted from patient to patient in highly contagious airborne droplets

Characteristics and pathogenesis: Small gm-rods; **filamentous hemagglutinin (FHA) capsule and pili; pertussis toxin (works via ADP-ribosylation) and tracheal cytotoxin, extra cytoplasmic cAMP**

Diagnosis: Culture on **Bordet-Genou** agar

Treatment: erythromycin; *B. pertussis* vaccine

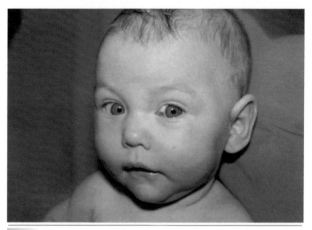

FIGURE 4.2   Clinical presentation of *Bordetella pertussis*. Not just a cute baby, examine the eyes. Severe coughing → conjunctival hemorrhaging.

BACTERIA

GRAM-NEGATIVE RODS (RESPIRATORY)—cont'd

History of present illness: 72 yo nursing home smoker on corticosteroids develops influenza-like symptoms of 2-week duration. Cough
is initially nonpurulent. After 1 week, the patient's symptoms worsen
with difficulty respiring. Patient is febrile to 39° C. Bilateral chest
pain and hemoptysis are present. She refuses treatment, loses consciousness, and is rushed to the ER. CXR shows a multilobar infiltrate
(Figure 4.3). Blood analysis shows increased LFTs, hyponatremia, and
hypophosphatemia. The patient expires. Most likely etiological agent:

Legionella pneumonia
Disease: Atypical pneumonia (similar to mycoplasma and influenza)
Characteristics and pathogenesis: Air conditioners in nursing homes
    are prime sites because the organism is airborne from water sources;
    immunosuppression, alcohol use, and smoking are risk factors
Diagnosis: Growth in **cysteine and iron** medium; **urine antigen test**
Treatment: erythromycin

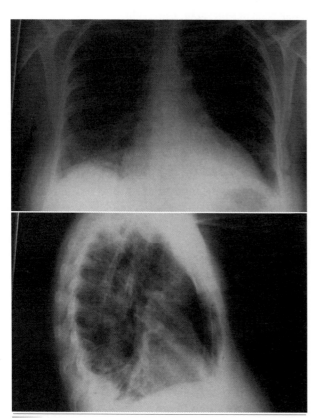

FIGURE 4.3 *Legionella pneumonia* on CXR.

BACTERIA

CHAPTER 5: GRAM-NEGATIVE RODS, (NOSOCOMIAL)

History of present illness: 26 yo patient with cystic fibrosis is status post appendectomy 2 days when she develops an infection at the wound site. The patient had been administered a third-generation cephalosporin. The wound is characterized by a specific musty odor and has a slightly green exudate. Dressing changes and antibiotic therapy seem to be futile until combination therapy is administered. Most likely etiological agent:

Pseudomonas aeruginosa
Disease: Wound and burn infections, corneal infections, pneumonia, osteomyelitis, opportunistic infections in patients with **CF**, immuno-compromised, nosocomial infections, and **malignant** otitis externa. Bad stuff: sepsis and endocarditis
Characteristics and pathogenesis: Normal flora of **colon**, strict **aerobe**; does not ferment glucose; does not reduce nitrates; **oxidase** +; exotoxin-like *C. diptheriae;* (**ADP-ribosylation**)
Diagnosis: Clinical, characteristic odor, green secretions in wounds; abscess by production of **pyocyanin, pyoverdin**
Treatment: Resistance high, multidrug regimen (e.g., ciprofloxacin, clinamycin, metronidazole)

♦   ♦   ♦

History of present illness: 23 yo immunocompromised patient, 3 days post-surgery presents with high temperature and decreasing blood pressure. Accompanying symptoms include difficulty respiring, nausea (no vomiting), and profuse diarrhea. PE reveals an acute ulcerative gingivitis and bronchi bilaterally. Most likely etiological agent:

Bacteroides fragilis
Disease: Intraabdominal sepsis (abscesses, peritonitis), oral infections, aspiration pneumonia
Characteristics and pathogenesis: Anaerobic gram negative, **no LPS** but capsule allows virulence. No exotoxin
Diagnosis: Grow on complex media
Treatment: metronidazole

CHAPTER 6: GRAM-NEGATIVE RODS, ZOONOTIC

History of present illness: 12 yo adolescent tending cows in rural Uzbekistan develops night sweats, malaise, chills, and mild headache. What is most peculiar is the presence of undulating fevers with temperatures ranging from 40° C to 36.5° C over a 1-day period. On PE, the patient is noted to have splenomegaly, hepatomegaly, and vertebral tenderness of L3 to L5. Patient is "not himself," as told by friends. Most likely etiological agent:

Brucella melitensis
Disease: Brucellosis, influenza-like syndrome with **undulating fever** (higher during day, lower at night); lymphadenopathy, hepatosplenomegaly, without ulcers or buboes
Characteristics and pathogenesis: Facultative intracellular gram-negative rods found in farm animals and transmitted by nonpasteurized milk products through skin; organisms localize in **reticuloendothelial system** (i.e., macrophages → granulomas)
Diagnosis: Serology; clinical diagnosis
Treatment: gentamycin, aminoglycosides, animal vaccination

♦   ♦   ♦

History of present illness: 14th century patient is transported by time portal to the present. 36 yo presents with severe swelling bilaterally of the submandibular nodes. Patient has had fever to 40° C and difficulty respiring for 3 weeks. People in his neighborhood have died and there is mass chaos. PE demonstrates hepatomegaly and bronchi bilaterally in the lungs. Coagulation times are high. Most likely etiological agent:

Yersinia pestis, **plague**

BACTERIA

BACTERIA

History of present illness: 15 yo complains of right lower quadrant pain for 1 week, an inability to eat, vomitus for 2 days, and no diarrhea. Patient is extremely tender at McBurney's point and has a positive Rovsing's sign and other signs of peritonitis. Surgery reveals a completely normal appendix. Most likely etiological agent:

Yersinia pseudotuberculosis: Mesenteric adenitis, pseudoappendicitis syndrome

Disease: Plague: fever, pneumonia, hemorrhage, shock, **DIC** via hematogenous dissemination

Characteristics and pathogenesis: Facultative **intracellular** gram-negative rods with **bipolar** stain; found in **prairie dogs** in the United States; most cases in the present day found in urban **Southeast Asia**; transmitted by respiratory droplets; organism spreads to regional lymph nodes; enlarged tender **buboes,** hemorrhages under the skin → blackish discoloration → hence the name "black death"

Diagnosis: Immunofluorescence, clinical diagnosis

Treatment: aminoglycoside, gentamycin; public health measures when outbreaks occur

CHAPTER 7: MYCOBACTERIAL RODS

History of present illness: 36 yo homeless woman complains of fever of 2 week duration, hemoptysis of 1 week duration, night sweats, and weight loss. Other people in close proximity have reported similar symptoms in the past. Patient is unable to walk or to give a coherent medical history. PE shows ronchi and rales found in all lobes of both lungs. Some nuchal rigidity is present. CXR is equally impressive with diffuse infiltrates throughout the field (Figures 7.1–7.3). Most likely etiological agent:

Mycobacterium tuberculosis (Figure 7.4)

Disease: Tuberculosis: fever, night sweats, cough, hemoptysis, weight loss

Characteristics and pathogenesis: Obligate intracellular aerobe; **mycolic acids** in cell wall allow organism to be acid-fast; **waxD** is the active ingredient in **Freund's adjuvant; cord factor** (for **virulence**), **granuloma** or **tubercle formation** → **caseous necrosis, fibrosis; Ghon-Sachs focus** on CXR (with perihilar lymph nodes— **Ghon-Sachs complex**); secondary TB (reactivation) infects **upper lobe (obligate aerobe)** of lung; liquefaction of lung and multiorgan involvement—cervical LN: (**scrofula**) (Figure 7.5), spine: (**Pott's disease**); miliary TB; older, immunocompromised, and malnourished adult at risk

Diagnosis: PPD test for immune response (prior exposure); immuno-compromised have weak response, therefore treat AIDS patients with low threshold; sputum exam three times with **acid-fast stain; NaOH** concentrate on **Lowenstein-Jensen medium** to culture organism (takes forever, 3 to 8 weeks); **niacin production**

Treatment: Resistance high; use multidrug regimen: prolonged, multiple Tx (e.g., isoniazid, rifampin, pyrazinamide, ethambutol); BCG vaccine used in some countries, efficacious primarily for severe pediatric sequelae and less for pulmonary TB

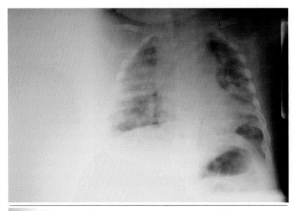

FIGURE 7.1 CXR of tuberculosis. © *Dr. Roger Smalligan.*

MYCOBACTERIAL RODS—cont'd

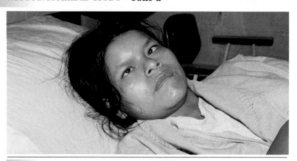

FIGURE 7.2 Clinical presentation of a TB patient.
© Dr. Roger Smalligan.

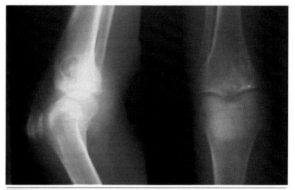

FIGURE 7.3 Tuberculosis infection of the bone.
© Dr. Roger Smalligan.

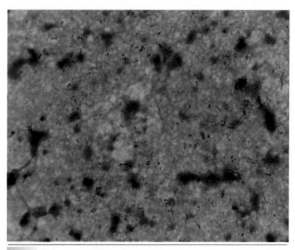

FIGURE 7.4 *Mycobacterium tuberculosis.*

MYCOBACTERIAL RODS—cont'd

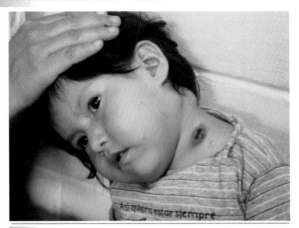

FIGURE 7.5   Scrofula. © *Dr. Roger Smalligan.*

History of present illness: 23 yo man from the Sudan complains of skin deformation of 3 years duration. PE reveals diffuse thickening of skin of the extremities, loss of sensation in these extremities, and hypopigmentation of the skin. The patient also exhibits loss of eyebrow hair, enlarged earlobes, and broadening of the nose. Most likely etiological agent:

Mycobacterium leprae

Disease: Leprosy: infects skin; superficial nerves in extremities (**lower** body temperature); destructive lesions; and neuropathy

Two types:

Tuberculoid: **Good** T-cell response, **granulomas, positive** lepromin skin test, not contagious; positive Mitsuda test, HLA-DR 2,3 association

Lepromatous: **Poor** T-cell response, lots of organisms, foamy histiocytes, **negative** lepromin skin test eyebrow alopecia, hypopigmentation, bone resorption, skin thickening, anesthesia, disfigurement; **negative Mitsuda test; HLA-DQ1** association

Characteristics and pathogenesis: obligate aerobe, facultative intracellular organisms, acid-fast rod that replicates intracellularly. Greatest worldwide prevalence in **Brazil, India,** and **Sudan.** Mouse footpad and armadillo **to culture organism (difficult to grow) currently grown in artificial culture; transmission difficult;** prolonged contact with patients, skin or aerosol transmission

Diagnosis: Clinical diagnosis, previous tests

Treatment: dapsone, rifampin

CHAPTER 8: GRAM-POSITIVE RODS

History of present illness: 64 yo s/p renal transplant patient on immunosuppressive therapy develops nuchal rigidity and fever to 39° C after eating cheese. Patient subsequently goes into shock. Blood tests reveal the following organism:

Listeria monocytogenes
Disease: Listeriosis with **neonatal** septicemia and meningitis; abscesses, granulomas, lymphadenitis also prevalent; abortion or premature delivery; transmitted to newborns and immunocompromised humans from animal feces or **unpasteurized milk and cheese**
Characteristics and pathogenesis: Facultative intracellular anaerobes; **nonsporeforming**, tumbling motility; **only gram positive with LPS**; infects **monocytes** and → granulomas; **listeriolysin O** used to make holes in attacked cells
Diagnosis: Gram-positive rods, beta hemolysis
Treatment: ampicillin

◆   ◆   ◆

History of present illness: 2 yo nonimmunized child presents with pharyngitis of 3 day duration and a **gray, fibrinous membrane** in the posterior oropharynx (Figure 8.1). The patient currently has apparent difficulty breathing. On PE, there is an irregular pulse along with tachycardia. The lungs are clear. A swelling of the neck from inflammation has caused a **"bull-neck"** appearance (Figure 8.2). Most likely etiological agent:

Corynebacterium diphtheriae (Figure 8.3)
Disease: Diphtheria: inflammation of posterior pharynx, myocarditis, recurrent laryngeal nerve palsy
Characteristics and pathogenesis: Gram-positive rod, **nonsporeforming**, nonmotile, club-shaped organism with K-antigen for antiphagocytic activity and exotoxin for ADP ribosylation of elongation factor-2 to inhibit host cell protein synthesis; tox gene required for toxicity
Diagnosis: Three tests: **Schick's, Loeffler, tellurite** cultures, and **Albert's** stain
Treatment: equine diphtheria antitoxin, penicillin

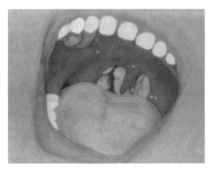

FIGURE 8.1
Fibrinous membrane in the posterior oropharynx.

GRAM-POSITIVE RODS—cont'd

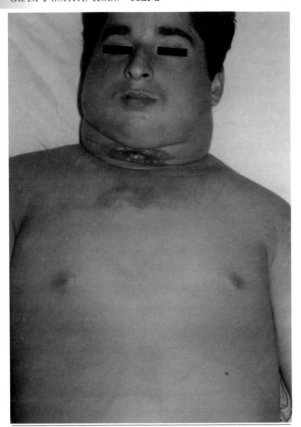

FIGURE 8.2   "Bull neck" appearance of diphtherial infection.

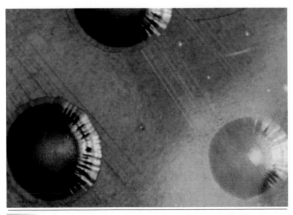

FIGURE 8.3   Respiratory paralysis with clostridium infection.

GRAM-POSITIVE RODS—cont'd

History of present illness: 42 yo cattle rancher presents to the ER with an infected laceration on the left lower extremity. The patient is discharged but returns with a malignant pustule at the wound site that appears necrotic by its dark color. The patient rapidly decompensates. Cavitary lesions and pulmonary infarcts are observed on radiography. Patient subsequently expires, in shock within 24 hours. Most likely etiological agent:

Anthrax: *Bacillus anthracis*
Disease: Woolsorters' disease: pulmonary anthrax; infection by **spores** on animal products (skins and hides) through skin and in the gastrointestinal and respiratory tracts
Characteristics and pathogenesis: Large with square ends; **nonmotile**; aerobic, **spore-forming** with exotoxin; **antiphagocytic capsule** made of **d-glutamate; tripartite anthrax toxin:** protective antigen, lethal factor, edema factor
Diagnosis: Morphology and blood agar growth
Treatment: penicillin

♦　　♦　　♦

History of present illness: 12 yo boy presents with abdominal pain, diarrhea without blood for **4 hours** and is afebrile. Patient had been eating **fried rice** at school, which had been warmed several times. A blood culture reveals no staphylococcus, but rather the following organism:

Bacillus cereus
Disease: GI infection and vomiting
Characteristics and pathogenesis: Spore-forming, heat stable toxin; motile; no capsule; **heat-labile** enterotoxin; **short** incubation period with little or **no** fever, typified by **vomiting**
Diagnosis: Clinical
Treatment: Symptomatic treatment

Gram-Positive Rods—cont'd

History of present illness: 32 yo man presents with swelling and
erythema of the lower right extremity after stepping on a nail. The
wound site is apparently infected. The patient also has "stiff" muscles
that do not relax well. The patient has difficulty breathing and has an
unusual wry smile. The patient has never had any vaccinations or immu-
nizations. PE also reveals hyperreflexia. Most likely etiological agent:

Clostridium tetani (Figure 8.4)

Disease: Tetanus: muscle tetany; **risus sardonicus** ("joker smile");
exaggerated reflexes; respiratory failure

Characteristics and pathogenesis: Anaerobic, spore-forming, with
exotoxin; **spores** in soil enters the wound; tetanus toxin travels axon-
ally in CNS and blocks release of inhibitory **glycine** neurotransmitter

Diagnosis: Clinical

Treatment: tetanus **toxoid** first; antibiotics (e.g., penicillin) can also be
used; ventilatory support and muscle relaxants can be administered if
symptoms become severe

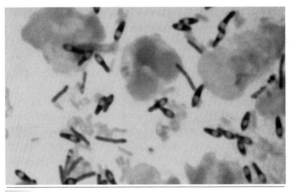

Figure 8.4 *Clostridium tetani.*

GRAM-POSITIVE RODS—cont'd

History of present illness: 23 yo patient presents with weakness of increasing severity for 2-day duration. Also noted are patientosis bilaterally, mydriasis, dysphagia, dysphonia, no urine output for 1 day, despite copious fluid intake and a palpated bladder to the periumbilical region. The patient had motor function in lower extremities the first day of illness, but now is apparently completely paralyzed. Noteworthy in the history is consumption of **canned green beans** in a bloated cannister 3 days earlier. Within 1 hour of admission, patient goes into respiratory arrest and is placed on a ventilator. Most likely etiological agent:

Clostridium botulinum (Figure 8.5)

Disease: Botulism: muscle paralysis and weakness, diplopia, respiratory failure if severe

    Wound botulism: spores in soil infect wound → release toxin

    Infant botulism: inadequate sterilization of canned foods; ingestion of spores in honey → **floppy baby syndrome**

Characteristics and pathogenesis: Anaerobic, spore-forming, preformed exotoxin spreads to nerves and **blocks Ach release**

Diagnosis: Clinical

Treatment: antitoxin; ventilatory support; penicillin is a bad idea: recommended since it releases more exotoxin from cells

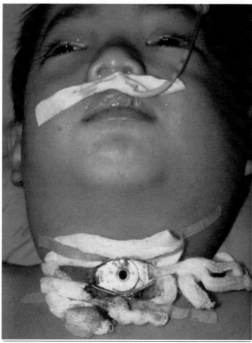

FIGURE 8.5 Respiratory paralysis with clostridium infection.

GRAM-POSITIVE RODS—cont'd

History of present illness: 18 yo soldier in Kosovo presents with large wound of the left lower extremity secondary to a grenade explosion. The patient has second- and third-degree wounds and numerous open lacerations where muscle and bone are exposed. Surrounding areas are characterized by severe edema, crepitus, and bullous lesions with a dark fluid. The extremity in general has a bronze pallor; patient is decompensating rapidly. Most likely etiological agent:

Clostridium perfringens (Figure 8.6)
Disease: Gas gangrene: dirty wounds and burns; food poisoning; **crepitus** from gas production; also hemolysis

Characteristics and pathogenesis: Anaerobic, spore-forming, found as normal flora of colon and vagina; **alpha toxin;** lecithinase degrades cell membranes

Diagnosis: Cell morphology, culture of wound. Other miscellaneous tests: sugar fermentation and organic acid production

Treatment: Oxygen gas: hyperbaric treatment kills anaerobes; penicillin; surgical excision and débridement

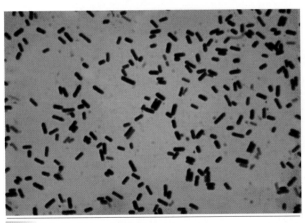

FIGURE 8.6 *Clostridum perfringens.*

Gram-Positive Rods—cont'd

History of present illness: 33 yo woman poststatus 5-day course of penicillin therapy develops diarrhea without blood. The patient's physicians administer ciprofloxacin to no avail, and her symptoms worsen. Overzealous gastroenterologists perform endoscopy on the patient, which reveals numerous small pseudomembranous colon plaques with mildly distended loops of bowel. Most likely etiological agent:

Clostridium difficile (Figure 8.7)
Disease: *Pseudomembranous colitis*
Characteristics and pathogenesis: Use of Abx (clindamycin, ampicillin, cephalosporins) kills normal flora and allows overgrowth; exotoxin A (diarrhea), exotoxin B (damage to colonic mucosa) (Figure 8.8)
Diagnosis: Toxin in stool
Treatment: vancomycin

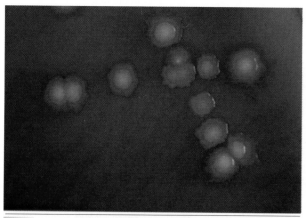

FIGURE 8.7 *Clostridium difficile.*

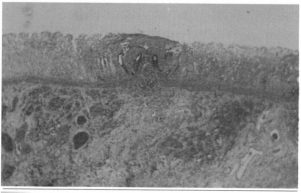

FIGURE 8.8 *Pseudomembranous colitis.*

CHAPTER 9: GRAM-NEGATIVE COCCI

History of present illness: 23 yo college student presents with nuchal rigidity, fever to 40° C, severe headache, and general malaise. A petechial rash in extremities and multiple hermorrhagic skin lesions are noted. Patient has a BP of 80/40. A CBC shows a WBC count of 14,000 and platelets of 50,000. Most likely etiological agent:

Neisseria meningitidis (Figures 9.1–9.2)

Disease: Meningitis: nuchal rigidity, fever, headache, photophobia; general meningococcemia: petechial rash fever, arthralgia, associated with patients with **C5-9** complement deficiency; **Waterhouse-Friderichsen syndrome:** fever, purpura, DIC, adrenal insufficiency from **bilateral adrenal** hemorrhage, shock, death

Characteristics and pathogenesis: Gram-negative diplococci in kidney-bean shape, **polysaccharide capsule, endotoxin (LPS);** IgA protease oxidase +; grows in **Thayer-Martin** medium, **chocolate** agar

Diagnosis: Increased PMN cells; gram stain of organism in CSF; ferments **maltose**; positive **latex agglutination** test

Treatment: ceftriaxone (penetrates CNS) vaccine is available.

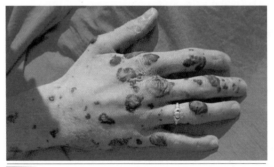

FIGURE 9.1 Petechial rash of *Neisseria meningitidis.*

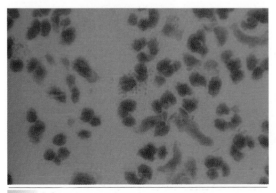

FIGURE 9.2 Diplococci of *Neisseria meningitidis.*

BACTERIA

GRAM-NEGATIVE COCCI—cont'd

History of present illness: 22 yo sexually active woman presents with bilateral lower abdominal pain with varying intensity for 4 weeks. Patient has had no diarrhea, vomiting, or dysuria and has severe cervical motion tenderness. A yellow discharge is noted from an obtained cervical specimen. Most likely etiological agent:

Neisseria gonorrhoeae

♦   ♦   ♦

History of present illness: 1-week-old baby is irritable and cries without ceasing. Patient apparently grabs at his eyes. Examination of the eyes reveals an erythema of the epicanthal and conjunctival regions of both eyes. Both lids have a yellow crusty exudate.

Neisseria gonorrhoeae (Figures 9.3–9.4)
Disease:
   Male: **urethritis**, dysuria, penile discharge; progresses to
      epididymitis and prostatitis, septic arthritis
   Female: cervicitis, PID, tubo-ovarian abscess; all lead to infertility;
      perihepatitis **(Fitz-Hugh–Curtis syndrome)**, septic arthritis
   Newborns: ophthalmia neonatorum
Characteristics and pathogenesis: Gram-negative cocci in kidney-bean
   shape but **no** capsule, **pili/fimbriae; endotoxin (LPS: lipopoly-
   saccharide)**, IgA protease, grows in **Thayer-Martin** medium,
   chocolate agar
Diagnosis: Does **NOT** ferment maltose; diplococci in PMN cells, usually
   a clinical diagnosis
Treatment: ceftriaxone, erythromycin eye drops; cream at birth for
   newborns; **no** vaccine (no capsule)

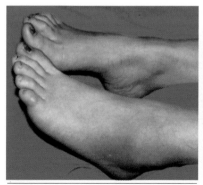

FIGURE 9.3 Septic arthritis.

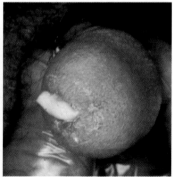

FIGURE 9.4 Penile discharge from *Neisseria* infection.

CHAPTER 10: GRAM-POSITIVE COCCI

History of present illness: 3-week-old child presents with an indurated, erythematous rash around the umbilicus, progressively spreading since birth. Temperatures have been consistently around 39° C the previous week. Patient cries continually, and the abdomen is severely distended. Most likely etiological agent:

Staphylococcus aureus (Figure 10.1)
Disease: Skin infections: omphalitis (as previously described), impetigo, cellulitis, erysipelas, abscess, furuncle, carbuncle (Figure 10.2)

◆   ◆   ◆

History of present illness: 25 yo woman presents with fever, vomiting, diarrhea of 2 days duration, and diffuse erythematous rash. Most likely etiological agent:

<u>S</u>taphylococcus aureus
Disease: <u>T</u>oxic shock syndrome: Shock and organ failure
           <u>A</u>cute endocarditis: Destructive (versus nondestructive with
                S. viridans and *S. faecalis*) (Figure 10.3)
           <u>P</u>neumonia: Damaging process, cavitations, empyema,
                effusions (Figure 10.4)
           <u>F</u>ood poisoning: 2- to 5-hr onset; **short** incubation period,
                with **little or no** fever; typified by **vomiting;** preformed
                toxin in sliced meats, custards, cream fillings
spells <u>S-T-A-P-F</u>: *Staphylococcus aureus*

<u>O</u>ther <u>B</u>ad stuff:
           <u>B</u>acteremia/sepsis: hematogenous spread
           <u>O</u>steomyelitis/septic joints/arthritis: hematogenous and
                traumatic spread
Characteristics and pathogenesis:
    <u>A</u>lpha toxin (lecithinase): Skin necrosis; hemolysis
    Protein <u>A</u>: Binds IgG-Fc, blocks opsonization and complement fixation
    <u>C</u>oagulase: Activates prothrombin
    <u>E</u>nterotoxin: Vomiting, diarrhea, toxin released in intestines
    <u>E</u>xfoliatin: Scalded skin, burn victims
    <u>F</u>ibrinolysin: Fibrin clot lysis
    <u>H</u>yaluronidase: Proteoglycan degradation
    <u>H</u>emolysin: Destroys RBCs, PMNs, MOs, platelets
    <u>L</u>eukocidin: destroys WBCs
    <u>T</u>SST-1: tampon use, wounds
AACEE FHHLT ("scrape your knee on asphalt" → staph abscess)
Diagnosis: Gram-positive cocci in grapelike clusters; **catalase positive;**
    β-hemolysis, coagulase positive, Yellow (Au) pigment
Treatment: Resistance common via β-lactamase; therefore
    methicillin, nafcillin, dicloxacillin; **MRSA:** (methicillin-resistant
    S. aureus): vancomycin

GRAM-POSITIVE COCCI—cont'd

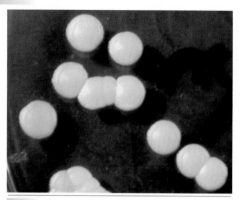

FIGURE 10.1   *Staphylococcus aureus.*

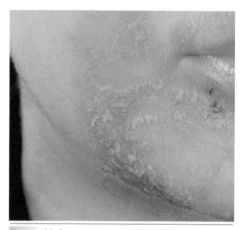

FIGURE 10.2   Dermatologic staph infection.

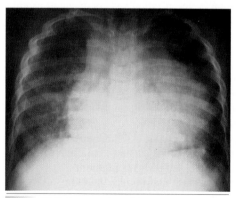

FIGURE 10.3   Acute endocarditis. © *Dr. Roger Smalligan.*

GRAM-POSITIVE COCCI—cont'd

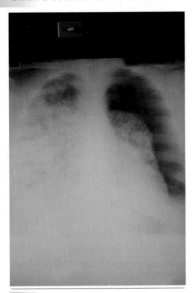

FIGURE 10.4 Staph pneumonia.
          © Dr. Roger Smalligan.

History of present illness: 59 yo man is hospitalized for 3 weeks for hip fracture. He develops chest pain, tachycardia, and severe pain and tenderness at site of hip replacement. Most likely etiological agent:

S. epidermidis
Disease: Endocarditis, especially with damaged or prosthetic heart valves; osteomyelitis, often nosocomial; also associated with IV catheters, often found as blood culture contaminant

♦   ♦   ♦

History of present illness: 35 yo woman presents with suprapubic pain for 3 days, dysuria, and fever. Most likely etiological agent:

S. saprophyticus
Disease: Community-acquired UTI
Diagnosis: Coagulase-negative staphylococcus
    S. epidermidis: novobiocin **sensitive**
    S. saprophyticus: novobiocin **resistant**
Treatment: As previously described

GRAM-POSITIVE COCCI—cont'd

History of present illness: 14 yo boy presents with fever to 39° C, chills, and erythematous posterior pharynx, with severely swollen strawberry-colored tonsils for the previous 3 days.

History of present illness: 12 yo girl presents with fever and polyarticular joint pain of 1-week. Patient had initial symptoms of a sore throat, which resolved within 2 days. On PE, it is noted that the patient has tachycardia.

β-hemolytic—Group A
SSTRePtococcus pyogenes
Disease:

<u>S</u>kin and soft tissue infections: Impetigo, cellulitis, necrotizing fasciitis, erysipelas: (Figure 10.5)

<u>S</u>carlet fever: Centrifugal rash, erythrogenic toxin, slap cheeks, strawberry tongue (Figure 10.6)

<u>T</u>oxic shock syndrome: Similar to staphylococcus infection

<u>R</u>heumatic fever: Fever, myocarditis, polyarthritis, chorea, subcutaneous nodules, erythema marginatum rash. Mitral valve disease follows pharyngitis as antibodies to bacteria cross react with joint and heart antigens

<u>P</u>haryngitis: "Classic strep throat," erythema, tonsillar swelling and exudate, fever

Acute glomerulonephritis: Hypertension, hematuria, edema of face and ankles. Follows both pharyngitis and skin infections. Same antibody cross-reactivity as previously described; deposits in the glomerular basement membrane

Characteristics and pathogenesis:

<u>M</u> protein: Inhibits phagocytosis

Ig<u>A</u> protease: Self-explanatory

<u>S</u>treptokinase: Converts plasminogen to plasmin; dissolves fibrin clots

<u>F</u> Protein: Adherence-fibronectin

<u>E</u>rythrogenic toxin: Scarlet fever

Streptolysin <u>S</u> and <u>O</u>: Results in β-**hemolysis**

C<u>5</u>a peptidase: Inhibits complement

<u>H</u>yaluronidase: Degrades proteoglycans

MAS FEO que 5 HigadoS ("More ugly than 5 livers in Spanish.") [Come up with your own mnemonics if you have a problem with these.]

Diagnosis: Clinical diagnosis; rapid strep test; blood agar to view hemolysis; sensitive to bacitracin

Treatment: penicillin (first choice), erythromycin, vancomycin

GRAM-POSITIVE COCCI—cont'd

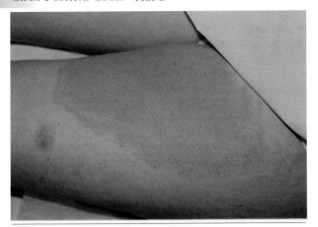

FIGURE 10.5 Strep cellulitis.

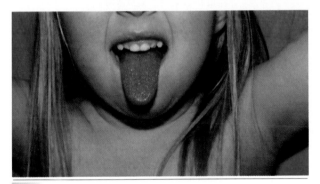

FIGURE 10.6 Strawberry tongue of scarlet fever.

GRAM-POSITIVE COCCI—cont'd

Other Strep:

ß-hemolytic—Group B

Streptococcus agalactiae: **Neonatal meningitis**/sepsis, **bacitracin resistant, nonhemolytic or gamma-hemolytic**

Streptococcus viridians: **Subacute endocarditis,** caries, nonbile soluble, optochin **resistant**

Streptococcus pneumoniae: **Lobar pneumonia, adult meningitis,** (Figure 10.7), bile soluble, optochin **sensitive**

Streptococcus faecalis: **Subacute endocarditis, UTI, growth in NaCl**

Streptococcus bovis: **Urinary tract infection (UTI), no growth in NaCl**

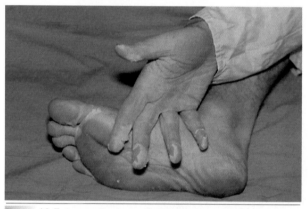

FIGURE 10.7 Dermatologic manifestations of toxic shock syndrome.

CHAPTER 11: SPIROCHETES

History of present illness: 10 yo child was in the woods helping her father shoot deer when she noticed a bite on her leg. Approximately 12 days later, she notices a circular rash with a clear center at the site of the bite. The area is erythematous and swollen. In addition, she is having chest pain, as well as joint pain in all four extremities for the last 2 weeks. On PE, a drooping mouth is noticed. Most likely etiological agent:

Borrelia burgdorferi

Disease: Lyme Disease: (1) **Erythema chronicum migrans** (Figure 11.1): circular red rash with clear center at bite, (2) "Itis": myocarditis, pericarditis, meningitis, **arthritis in large** joints, (3) Neuro: CNS involvement, neuropathy

Characteristics and pathogenesis: Large organism; spiral morphology; found in **white-footed mouse** and transmitted via deer tick *(Ixodes)* to humans (Figure 11.2)

Diagnosis: Darkfield microscopy with Giemsa stain; ELISA antibody

Treatment: doxycycline

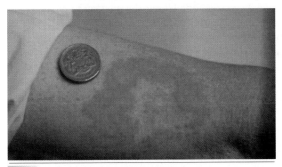

FIGURE 11.1 Erythema chronicum migrans.

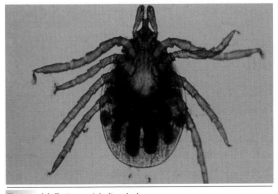

FIGURE 11.2 Deer tick *(Ixodes)*.

SPIROCHETES—cont'd

History of present illness: 52 yo man from Telluride, Colorado, complains of fever that has come and gone for the last 2 weeks. Also, chills, malaise, other influenza-like symptoms have peculiarly resolved and then resumed three times in the last 6 days. Patient is not immunocompromised and is not on medication. Most likely etiological agent:

Borrelia hermsii or *Borrelia recurrentis*
Disease: Relapsing fever: fever and chills; can progress to multiorgan involvement
Characteristics and pathogenesis: Large organism with spiral morphology, antigenic variation via **(variable major protein)** is cause of relapses in fever
Diagnosis: blood smears (Giemsa stain) show large spirochetes.
Treatment: doxycycline

◆   ◆   ◆

History of present illness: 35 yo sewage worker, who was swimming in the underground drainage system in New York the previous week, complains of fever, chills, headache, and fatigue for the last 24 hours. He has not been able to think clearly and wonders what the yellow tinge around his tongue could be. On PE, patient has mild nuchal rigidity. Blood work reveals elevated LFTs and BUN/Cr levels. Most likely etiological agent:

Leptospira interrogans
Disease: leptospirosis: acute febrile illness; symptoms similar to meningitis. **Weil's** disease (infectious jaundice, Figure 11.3): **h**epatorenal failure, **h**emorrhage, **h**eavy **h**ead (mental status changes)
Characteristics and pathogenesis: tightly coiled organism penetrates abraded skin via contaminated food, water, or by urine of infected rats, livestock, pets. Sewage workers and farmers are at the greatest risk. Lipopolysaccharide in outer membrane
Diagnosis: Tightly coiled spirochetes by **Darkfield microscopy** (Figure 11.4)
Treatment: penicillin, doxycycline

SPIROCHETES—cont'd

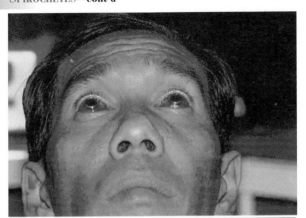

FIGURE 11.3 Jaundice secondary to leptospirosis.

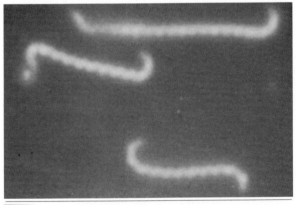

FIGURE 11.4 Tightly coiled leptospira.

Spirochetes—cont'd

History of present illness: 36 yo sexually active man complains of a painless lesion on his penis. On PE, the ulcer is indurated and well-circumscribed; bilateral inguinal lymph nodes are palpable. No other abnormalities are noted. The patient is given appropriate medication and leaves. After 2 months, the patient returns stating that he forgot to take his medication, but the ulcer healed anyway. He now complains of a maculopapular rash on the oral mucosa and soles of his feet. Most likely etiological agent:

Treponema pallidum: (Figure 11.5) Secondary syphilis
Disease: Congenital syphilis: Transmitted to fetus **after** first trimester, causing death or congenital abnormalities
  Primary syphilis: Nontender chancre; highly infectious; symptoms begin 6 weeks after infection; resolve 6 weeks after initial symptoms
  Secondary syphilis: Condyloma latum; lesions on palms, soles, **oral mucosa. Noninfectious stage is 6 weeks** after primary syphilis; symptoms can begin as spirochetes disseminate to organs (bacterial sepsis) (hepatitis/nephritis); **66%** resolve in **6** weeks; 33% progress to **tertiary** stage (alopecia)
  Tertiary syphilis: Tabes dorsalis (posterior column or dorsal root damage); bone and skin granulomas (benign **gummas**); aortic aneurysms; vascular infarcts; neurosyphilis. These symptoms begin 6 years later.
  Characteristics and pathogenesis: Thin-walled, flexible, tightly spiraled rods
Diagnosis: RPR/ VDRL to screen, **FTA-ABS** for definitive diagnosis
Treatment: penicillin

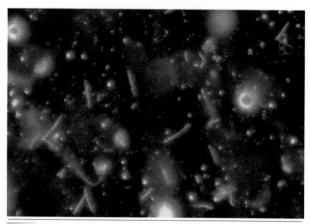

Figure 11.5 *Treponema pallidum.*

VIRUSES

CHAPTER 12: DNA-ENVELOPED VIRUSES

History of present illness (1): Newborn presents with IUGR (intrauterine growth retardation), jaundice, hepatosplenomegaly, thrombocytopenia, and encephalitis with microcephaly. In addition, the patient exhibits seizures and focal neurological signs.

◆   ◆   ◆

History of present illness (2): 65 yo immunocompromised patient, status post renal transplant presents with sharp, spiking pyrexia with elevated LFTs. Patient has difficulty respiring. CXR and PE reveal a serious pneumonitis. Additionally, patient complains of vision problems and blood in the stool.

(β):Cytomegalovirus (CMV)
Disease: Cytomegalic **inclusion body disease** in infants (**microcephaly,** deafness, second leading cause of mental retardation behind rubella). Immunocompromised and renal transplant patients: disseminated CMV septicemia, pneumonitis, **CMV retinitis,** hepatitis, GI ulceration and hemorrhage.
Characteristics and pathogenesis: Envelope +, double-stranded, linear DNA transmitted by all body fluids (e.g., oropharynx) → CNS, kidneys, across placenta, especially during third trimester, organ transplantation (immunocompromised). Remains latent in **leukocytes.**
Diagnosis: CPE, "owl's eye" nuclear inclusions, **Paul-Bunnel** test is **negative** versus EBV
Treatment: ganciclovir

◆   ◆   ◆

History of present illness: 23 yo presents with fever, pharyngitis, and lymphadenopathy lasting for 2 weeks. He wonders whether this is secondary to kissing his first girlfriend. PE reveals slight hepatosplenomegaly. CXR is clear. A Paul-Bunnel test is positive.

(γ):Epstein Barr (EBV)
Disease: Mononucleosis: Classic **triad** of fever, pharyngitis, and lymphadenopathy; associated with **Burkitt's lymphoma** in East Africa
Characteristics and pathogenesis: Envelope +, double-stranded, linear DNA transmitted via saliva to oropharynx epithelium → cervical lymph nodes → viremia in blood → liver and spleen → active latency in **B-lymphocytes**
Diagnosis: Paul-Bunnel/mono-spot (heterophile) test: **positive**
Treatment: No drug, no vaccine, supportive treatments

VIRUSES

DNA-Enveloped Viruses—cont'd

History of present illness: 43 yo male presents with tingling, itching, and burning sensation on the oral mucosa. A **gingival stomatitis** is diagnosed. After 5 days, painful **"cold sores"** develop. A cluster of vesicles (blisters) on the perioral skin rupture to form lesions. These are now **crusting** when the patient asks for medication.

(α) **Herpes simplex virus type I (HSV I)** Figures 12.1 and 12.2

Disease: Oral sores (herpes **labialis**) facial lessons, gingivostomatitis, **keratoconjunctivitis** → blindness in infants

Characteristics and pathogenesis: Envelope +, double-stranded, linear DNA, envelope generated from nuclear membrane; transmitted by saliva or direct contact, "stored," hides in axons (i.e., ganglial latency mechanism via the **LAT:** latency associated transcript)

Diagnosis: Via cytopathogenic effect (CPE) in cell culture, **Tzanck** smear has giant cells

Treatment: acyclovir for **encephalitis,** avoidance of sunlight; no vaccines currently available

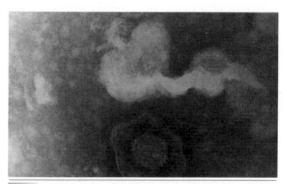

Figure 12.1 Herpes virus at high magnification.

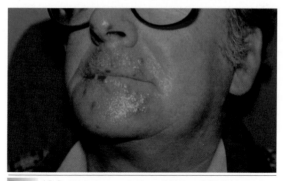

Figure 12.2 Clinical presentation of *Herpes labialis*.

DNA-Enveloped Viruses—cont'd

History of present illness: 34 yo man presents with shooting pains, numbness, aches felt in the **genital** region, back, buttocks, and left inner thigh. In addition, the patient has had fever, headaches, and **inguinal** lymphadenopathy. Patient returns 3 weeks later with erupting sores and blisters, with a few crusted lesions.

(α) Herpes simplex virus type II
Disease: Herpes **genitalis,** aseptic meningitis, and **neonatal** infection
Characteristics and pathogenesis: Envelope$^+$, double-stranded, linear DNA, envelope generated from nuclear membrane, transmitted by sexual contact in birth canal (avoid vaginal delivery of infected mothers → C-section). Virus starts as genital lesion and travels up axons to lumbar-sacral ganglia.
Diagnosis: CPE in cell culture, **Tzanck** smear shows giant cells
Treatment: acyclovir; no vaccines currently available

♦   ♦   ♦

History of present illness I: 36 yo immunocompromised woman presents with burning, shooting pain, as well as tingling and itching on the right side of the face, right neck, and upper chest. Rash and blisters have been present for 7 days. Patient is treated but returns 3 years later with pain in the region where the lesions healed (Figure 12.3).

History of present illness II: 4 yo presents with a small erythematous pruritic rash for 6 days. Clear blisters are found on a majority of the bumps of the maculopapular rash, as though dew drops on a petal. In certain regions, the rash has crusted or scabbed. A few sores appear on the **mucous membranes.** Patient is given medicine and sent home but returns 1 week later with persistent or recurrent vomiting, listlessness, personality changes (i.e., irritability and combativeness). Patient has had one incidence of loss of consciousness. It is noted that the mother administered **aspirin** in conjunction with the treatment given by the physician.

Varicella zoster (Figure 12.4)
Disease: Chicken pox in children (**Reye's** syndrome associated with aspirin use) → recurrence as zoster in adults (shingles, **unilateral** dermatome) with postherpetic neuralgia (PHN)
Characteristics and pathogenesis: Envelope +, double-stranded, linear DNA, transmitted as respiratory droplets → respiratory tract infected → viremia → liver → latency in **dorsal root sensory ganglia**→ PHN
Diagnosis: CPE in cell culture, 4x increase in antibody titer, fluorescence, **Tzanck smear;** rash follows dermatomal pattern
Treatment: No antivirals V216 varicella zoster immunoglobulin

DNA-ENVELOPED VIRUSES—cont'd

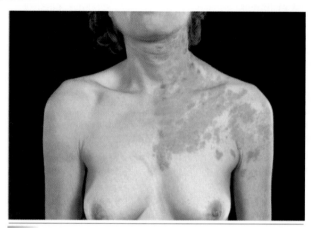

FIGURE 12.3 Dermatomal distribution of shingles.

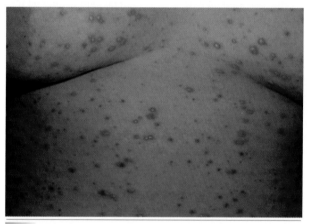

FIGURE 12.4 Clinical presentation of *Varicella zoster.*

CHAPTER 13: HEPATITIS TYPES ABCD

History of present illness: 45 yo IV drug user presents with jaundice, fatigue, abdominal pain, loss of appetite, and intermittent nausea and vomiting. PE reveals hepatomegaly and a yellow pallor. Blood work reveals elevated LFTs.

Hepatitis B virus
Disease: Hepatitis B hepatocellular cancer
Characteristics and pathogenesis: Hepadnavirus; envelope +, double-stranded, linear DNA, incomplete circular, three antigens (surface Ag: HBsAg, core Ag, e Ag)

	HBsAg surface antigen	HBsAb surface antibody	HBcAb core antibody
Complete recovery	−	+	+
Chronic carrier	+	−	+

Bloodborne disease transmitted via sex, IV drug use, response by CD8 T cells, antigen-antibody complexes can lead to autoimmune arthritis, rash, glomerulonephritis
Diagnosis: Clinical diagnosis; no cell culture, serologic tests
Treatment: Supportive treatment only, persistent infection versus hepatitis A (lifelong immunity); vaccine use has substantially decreased hepatitis B rates

VIRUSES

HEPATITIS TYPES ABCD—cont'd

Salient facts about other hepatitis viruses

Hepatitis A: **A**symptomatic, **A**cute, same clinical presentation as Hepatitis B (Figure 13.1)

Characteristics and pathogenesis: Picornavirus, RNA-nonenveloped virus, single-stranded + linear, no virion polymerase, fecal oral transmission → GI → liver, CD8 attack on liver, lifelong immunity, acute not chronic, shorter incubation period (3 to 4 weeks)

Diagnosis: IgM level

Treatment: No antiviral vaccine available

Hepatitis C: Flavivirus family, chronic, cirrhosis, carcinoma, carrier

Characteristics and pathogenesis: **RNA-enveloped virus, single-stranded** + RNA E^+ chronic carrier → hepatocellular carcinoma by CD8 T-cells, transmitted via blood (e.g., sexually, transfusions)

Treatment: α-interferon, no vaccine

Hepatitis D: Defective virus that requires concomitant infection with Hepatitis B

Treatment: Use hepatitis B surface antigen, **RNA-enveloped virus** single-stranded; RNA envelope$^+$

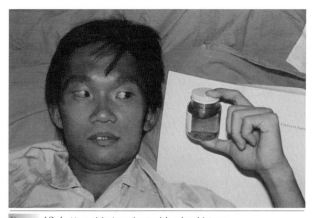

FIGURE 13.1 Hepatitis A patient with scleral icterus.

CHAPTER 14: DNA-Nonenveloped Viruses

History of present illness: 23 yo man living in military barracks presents with erythema and swelling of the posterior pharynx without exudate for the last 2 weeks. In addition to having a runny nose and eyes, bilateral conjunctiva are inflamed. Patient has self-medicated with Azithromycin to no avail. CXR shows a diffuse pneumonia.

Adenovirus (Figure 14.1)

Disease: Upper and lower respiratory infection, pneumonia, conjunctivitis, sarcomas, and hemorrhagic cystitis (rare)

Characteristics and pathogenesis: Envelope$^+$, double-stranded, linear DNA, nonenveloped, no virion polymerase, uses hemaggluttinin fibers for pathogenesis, used in molecular biology as a transfecting agent because of its rapid efficient entry; transmitted by respiratory droplets (fecal or oral) and with high prevalence in **military** or **university dormatory** close quarters

Diagnosis: Cytopathogenic effect (CPE) in culture; increase in Ab titer; no treatment; military vaccine available (enteric coated, live nonattenuated vaccine)

Treatment: Supportive

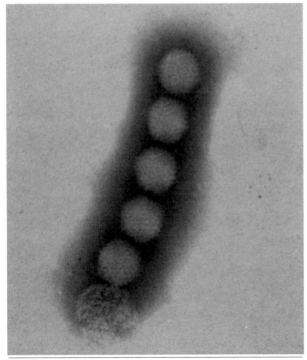

Figure 14.1 Adenovirus at high magnification.

DNA-NONENVELOPED VIRUSES—cont'd

History of present illness: 28 yo woman presents with warts on the external and internal wall of the vagina and the cervix, as well as perianally. She states that her husband had similar lesions on the tip of his penis and scrotum, as well as perianally. Patient has had no fever, rash, or other symptoms.

Papillomavirus

Disease: Human papillomavirus (HPV); **condylomata acuminata;** cervical cancer

Characteristics and pathogenesis: Envelope negative, double-stranded, linear DNA, circular supercoiled, no virion polymerase; first infects basal layer → skin/genital lesions → squamous epithelial cell growth → E6-7 genes of virus induce binding to p53 and other tumor suppressor genes → cervical cancer; HPV types **16,18** → cancer versus HPV **6,11** → warts only

Diagnosis: Koilocytosis: Cytoplasm vacuole in lesions, pap smear-colposcopy to observe abnormal cells; transformation to cancerous cells; pap smear screening the most effective anticancer intervention in twentieth century.

Treatment: Aldara (imiquimod) cream, trichloroacetic acid (TCA), podophyllin, cryosurgery (freezing), or electrocautery (burning)

DNA-NONENVELOPED VIRUSES—cont'd

History of present illness: 15 yo presents with mild cold symptoms, malaise, and a mild fever for 5 days, as well as a light red and lacy rash. Patient's face is intensely erythematous, especially on the cheeks, with a pale ring around the mouth (**"circumoral pallor"**) (Figure 14.2).

Parvovirus (B-19)
Disease: Erythema infectiosum, or "fifth's disease," with characteristic slapped cheek appearance, aplastic crisis in patients with sickle-cell anemia or other abnormalities of hemoglobin, **hydrops fetalis**
Characteristics and pathogenesis: Nonenveloped single-stranded, linear DNA, **smallest** of all viruses
Diagnosis: Clinical
Treatment: Supportive, no vaccine

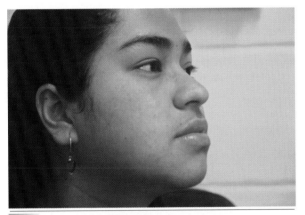

FIGURE 14.2 "Slapped cheek" of Parvovirus B-19 infection.
© *Dr. Roger Smalligan.*

VIRUSES

VIRUSES

CHAPTER 15: RNA-ENVELOPED VIRUSES

History of present illness: 34 yo man presents with fever of 39° C for 6 days, including shaking, chills, moderate muscle and joint ache, malaise, sweating, a dry cough, nasal congestion, sore throat, and headache.

Influenza virus A (epidemic: antigenic shift), B (major), or C (antigenic drift: mild disease/minor outbreaks)
Disease: Influenza, secondary bacterial pneumonia (Figure 15.1)
Characteristics and pathogenesis: Orthomyxovirus: Envelope+ single-stranded, linear-segmented RNA (therefore rearrangements); helical nucleocapsid; RNA polymerase in virion; two major Ag: hemagglutinin and neuraminidase (degrades mucin covering of mucosal epithelial cells → hemaglutinin sticks to sialic acid) on separate surface spikes (antigenic variation via reassortment of RNA segments results in epidemics, and therefore ineffectiveness of vaccines); transmitted by respiratory droplets; animal reservoir
Diagnosis: Clinical; can use hemadsorption or hemagglutination; Ab titer; no giant cells observed
Treatment: Supportive, amantadine and rimantadine, although not effective against influenza B or influenza C
New treatment in 2001: zanamivir, oseltamivir phosphate "rare", yearly vaccine in Fall

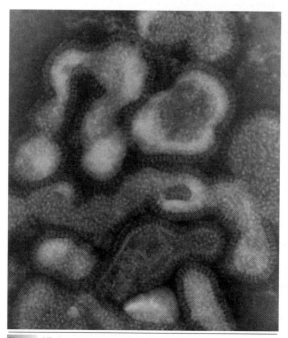

FIGURE 15.1 Influenza virus.

RNA-ENVELOPED VIRUSES—cont'd

History of present illness: Unvaccinated 5 yo child presents with high fever, rash, runny nose, watery eyes, and coughing for 1 week. Symptoms have not abated with antibiotic treatment. The rash is further characterized by an erythematous maculopapular appearance, which started at the head and spread **downward**.

Measles virus (Figure 15.2)

Disease: Measles: conjunctivitis (→ **photophobia**), Cough, Coryza (nasal discharge) Koplik's spots in mouth: red lesions with white dots → maculopapular rash on body → can progress to **subacute sclerosing panencephalitis** (SSPE)

Characteristics and pathogenesis: Paramyxoviruses: Envelope$^+$, single-stranded, linear, nonsegmented RNA($^-$), helical, RNA polymerase in virion budding. Transmitted by respiratory droplets → upper respiratory tract → lymph nodes → blood → skin, possible giant cell pneumonia and encephalitis

Diagnosis: Clinical, serology (if necessary)

Treatment: Supportive, MMR vaccine at 15 mo

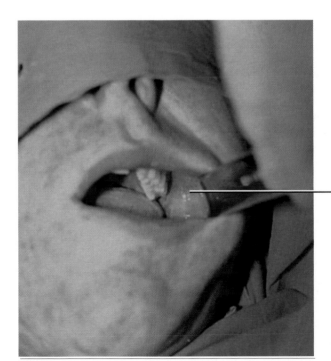

Koplik's spots

FIGURE 15.2 Clinical presentation of measles.

VIRUSES

RNA-ENVELOPED VIRUSES—cont'd

History of present illness: Unvaccinated 10 yo presents with fever, swelling, and tenderness of the salivary glands, particularly the left parotid gland. Swelling of the testicles is present, as well as focal neurologic deficits and nuchal rigidity.

Mumps virus

Disease: Mumps → **salivary gland** inflammation, fever, bilateral **orchitis,** can be complicated with encephalitis, meningitis, arthritis, kidney involvement, inflammation of the thyroid gland and breasts, deafness

Characteristics and pathogenesis: Envelope$^+$ single-stranded, linear, nonsegmented RNA($^-$), helical, RNA pol in virion budding; transmitted via respiratory droplets → upper respiratory tract → lymph nodes → bloodstream → other organs, swelling of **parotids**

Diagnosis: Clinical, hemadsorption, serology (if necessary)

Treatment: No antiviral therapy, MMR at 15 mo is most effective

◆   ◆   ◆

History of present illness: 2 yo child presents with hoarse, **barking** cough, high fever for 1 week. Symptoms began 1 week earlier as a simple cold. The patient is having difficulty breathing with a noisy **stridor.** Other family members are ill with colds and coughs. The child is uncomfortable and symptoms typically worsen at night.

Parainfluenza virus

Disease: Bronchiolitis in infants, laryngotracheobronchitis **(croup)** in children (barking cough, hoarse), cold in adults

Characteristics and pathogenesis: Envelope$^+$, single-stranded, linear, nonsegmented RNA($^-$), helical, RNA pol in virion budding, unlike influenza, hemagglutinin and neuramidase antigens are stable; transmitted via respiratory droplets → upper respiratory tract → **multinucleated giant cells** by viral fusion protein, a hallmark feature

Diagnosis: Clinical

Treatment: Initially, humidity and benadryl; oxygen and aerosolized epinephrine if severe; steroid decadron

RNA-ENVELOPED VIRUSES—cont'd

History of present illness: 3-month-old infant presents with tachypnea, tachycardia, fever to 39° C. The patient has had no vomiting, diarrhea, or hemoptysis. CXR shows a diffuse reticular pattern. Antibiotics have been ineffective the last few days and the patient appears to be worsening.

Respiratory syncytial virus (RSV)

Disease: Bronchiolitis and pneumonia in infants (#1 cause in infants < 6 mo old)

Characteristics and pathogenesis: Envelope$^+$, single-stranded + linear, nonsegmented RNA($^-$), helical, RNA polymerase in virion; unlike other paramyxoviruses, it has only a **fusion protein** in its surface spikes; therefore **no** hemagglutinin, transmitted via respiratory droplets → upper respiratory tract

Treatment: Aerosolized **ribavirin**, no vaccine

♦ ♦ ♦

History of present illness: 3 yo Malawian child presents with chest indrawing, tachypnea, fever to 38.5° C, and dry cough. Oxygen saturation is shown to be diminishing. CXR shows multiple fungal ball lesions. Blood work shows an unusual distribution and diminished white blood cell count from that which would be expected.

Human immunodeficiency virus (HIV)

Disease: Acquired immunodeficiency syndrome (AIDS): multiple disease presentations. You should know this virus already! Opportunistic infections include:
Pneumocystis pneumonia (PCP)
Kaposi's sarcoma
Thrush candidiasis
Mycobacterium (tuberculosis)
    All discussed separately later

Characteristics and pathogenesis: Retrovirus: E$^+$ two copies **(diploid),** single-stranded + RNA, RNA-dependent DNA polymerase, transmission by body fluids, sexual contact, IV drug abuse → CD4 T cells killed
Key proteins of pathogenesis:
gag → internal core proteins
pol → reverse transcriptase, integrase, viral protease (target of protease inhibitors)
env → glycoproteins (gp 120 → binds CD4 with gp 41)
tat → increase gene transcription to inhibit MHC I synthesis to evade host immune response

Diagnosis: ELISA, western blot

Treatment: AZT, protease inhibitors, retrovirals

VIRUSES

History of present illness: 32 yo man presents with an infected wound of the left lower extremity. He has difficulty respiring and is showing signs of neurologic involvement. He appears to have lost function of his facial muscles, and is **salivating** profusely. His history is notable in that his speech was slurred secondary to tongue **muscle paralysis** and that he was bitten by a dog 2 weeks earlier. His neighbors noted his hyperactivity, agitation, and confusion.

Rabies virus
Disease: Rabies, encephalitis, **hydrophobia**
Characteristics and pathogenesis: Rhabdovirus: E^+ helical nucleocapsid, single-stranded; RNA, RNA pol in virion zoonotic virus transmitted by animal bite → Ach receptor at neuron, up axon, replicates in brain → salivary glands→ symptoms
Diagnosis: Clinical, stain for the **negri** bodes
Treatment: No antiviral therapy, but 5-vaccine treatment in arm

♦   ♦   ♦

History of present illness: 6 yo non-immunized child presents with a fine, pink rash spreading from the forehead and face **downward.** The rash has lasted for 5 days. Occipital lymphadenopathy is present. The patient's mother has had similar symptoms with a fever, rash, and joint pain similar to arthritis.

Rubella virus
Disease: Rubella: German or 3-day measles, minor in adults and children, **fatal** in newborns; **developmental** malformations, **congenital rubella syndrome** (cardiac anomalies, cataracts; CNS—microcephaly)
Characteristics and pathogenesis: Togavirus—E^+ single-stranded + linear + RNA, no pol in virion, transmitted via nasopharynx → lymph and blood → skin; maculopapular rash, posterior auricular lymphadenopathy
Diagnosis: Increased **IgM** not IgG with amniocentesis in pregnant women. In adults, clinical diagnosis is sufficient, negative with cocksackie plaques, **no** CPE.
Treatment: Supportive, MMR vaccine

♦   ♦   ♦

Miscellaneous RNA-enveloped viruses
  Bunya viruses: E^+ single-stranded + RNA circular
    Hantavirus
    California encephalitis
  Filoviruses: E^+ single-stranded + RNA linear
    Ebola
    Hemorrhagic fever

CHAPTER 16: RNA-NONENVELOPED VIRUSES

History of present illness: 4 yo child has fever of 39° C, headache, and muscle aches. Mild sore throat, abdominal discomfort, and nausea are noted. The fever has been **biphasic**—present for 1 day, gone for 2 to 3 days, returning for 2 to 4 days more. A rash is revealed on PE: hand, foot, and mouth areas are affected.

Coxsackie virus (A or B)

Disease: Hand-foot-mouth disease (Figures 16.1 and 16.2), aseptic meningitis, **herpangina:** sore oropharynx-grey vesicles (A), pleurodynia-pleuritic chest pain (B), myocarditis: dilated cardiomyopathy (B), pericarditis (B)

Characteristics and pathogenesis: Picornavirus; fecal oral transmission, → oropharynx → GI → blood

Diagnosis: CPE in culture, Ab titer

Treatment: Supportive; no antiviral treatment or vaccine

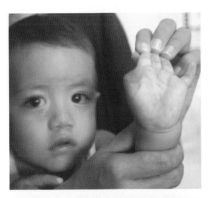

FIGURE 16.1
Hand-foot-mouth disease.
© *Dr. Roger Smalligan.*

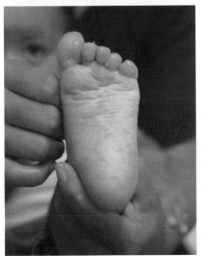

FIGURE 16.2
Hand-foot-mouth disease.
© *Dr. Roger Smalligan.*

VIRUSES

RNA-Nonenveloped Viruses—cont'd

History of present illness: 3 yo child presents with fever, nuchal rigidity, and apparent headache for 4 days. The patient suffers from malaise, cough, and diarrhea without blood. CSF tap reveals no bacteria and an elevated lymphocyte count.

Echovirus
Disease: Aseptic viral meningitis, upper respiratory infection (URIs), infantile diarrhea
Characteristics and pathogenesis: Type 30 echovirus most common for meningitis, fecal oral transmission
Diagnosis: Clinical diagnosis with CSF analysis; some use PCR
Treatment: Supportive

◆　　◆　　◆

History of present illness: 76 yo woman presents with abrupt onset of weakness in bilateral lower extremity muscles, accompanied by excessive fatigue, muscle and joint pain, and muscle atrophy. The patient's history is significant for not having had any vaccinations.

Poliovirus
Disease: Paralytic poliomyelitis, aseptic meningitis, **postpolio syndrome** is most common, because polio has been eradicated with the Salk and Sabin vaccines.
Characteristics and pathogenesis: Picornavirus: E (*2*) single-stranded + linear, no virion polymerase 3 serotypes, inclusion bodies, fecal oral transmission; → pharynx + GI → lymph → blood → CNS → meningitis (**anterior horn,** motor neurons) → cell death and paralysis (rare)
Diagnosis: Clinical, Ab titer, CPE in cell culture
Treatment: No antiviral; Sabin (live) and Salk (dead) vaccines widely used and efficacious

◆　　◆　　◆

History of present illness: 4 yo child presents with runny nose, sniffles, and no other significant findings. Patient has no nausea, vomiting, diarrhea, fever, chills.

Rhinovirus
Disease: Common cold
Characteristics and pathogenesis: Transmission by aerosol droplets, hand to nose (virus likes the cold environment of the nose 33° C; put your finger in your nose and you will see that it is colder there) → upper respiratory tract mucosa and conjunctiva (destroyed by **stomach acid,** therefore never a GI infection)
Diagnosis: Clinical
Treatment: Supportive, no antiviral, no vaccine (lots of antigenic variations)

RNA-NONENVELOPED VIRUSES—cont'd

History of present illness: 3 yo child presents with diarrhea of 1 week duration. There is no blood in the stool. The patient has been unable to retain any fluids. The buccal mucosa, oropharynx is dry, and moisture is virtually absent from the eyes. The patient has no nausea, vomiting, fever, or chills (Figure 16.3).

Reovirus/rotavirus (Figure 16.4)
Disease: Gastroenteritis; leading cause of fatal diarrhea and dehydration
Characteristics and pathogenesis: Nonenveloped double-stranded RNA, repeated parallel segments of RNA, fecal oral transmission, respiratory droplets, → lysis, no budding
Diagnosis: Clinical
Treatment: Fluid replacement, no antiviral, no vaccine

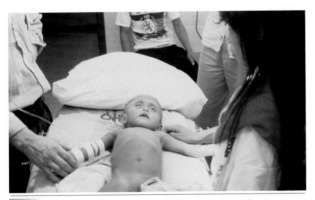

FIGURE 16.3 Clinical presentation of severe rotavirus infection: dehydration. © *Dr. Roger Smalligan.*

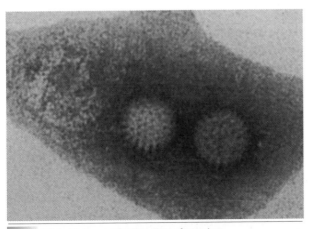

FIGURE 16.4 High magnification view of rotavirus.

VIRUSES

CHAPTER 17: Salient Facts About Arboviruses
(Arthropod-Borne)

Dengue fever virus (Figure 17.1)
- Flavivirus
- In the Carribean 2 types:
  (1) Classic dengue "breakbone fever" (joints and muscles) →
  influenza-like, **mild,** pain
  (2) Dengue hemorrhagic fever → like classic but leads to → shock
  and hemorrhage
- **10% fatal**

St. Louis encephalitis
- Flavivirus
- Mosquitoes from birds to humans
- Rural and **urban,** all over the United States
- **10% fatal**

Yellow fever virus
- Flavivirus (monkeys and humans)
- Mosquitoes **Aedes aegypti** → fever and jaundice, hence the name
  yellow fever → headache and myalgias
- Shock (12-14 day extrinsic incubation period) **councilman bodies**
  observed
- Live vaccine available

Eastern equine encephalitis virus
- **Alpha** virus
- Culex swamp mosquitoes from bird → humans and horses in
  Atlantic/Gulf coast
- Sudden onset of severe headache, nausea, vomiting, and coma
- **50% fatal**

Western equine encephalitis virus
- **Alpha** virus
- Mosquitoes, from birds to humans and horses
- **Rural** western United States
- Less severe than Eastern counterpart

SALIENT FACTS ABOUT ARBOVIRUSES (ARTHROPOD-BORNE)—cont'd

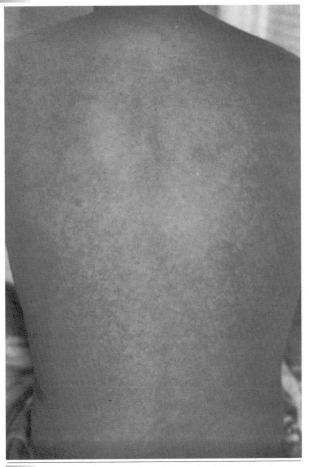

FIGURE 17.1 Clinical presentation of hemorrhagic Dengue rash.

VIRUSES

CHAPTER 18: ZEBRAS, ERADICATED VIRUSES, AND PRIONS

Small pox virus

Disease: Small pox (eradicated); maculopapular rash

Characteristics and pathogenesis: Pox viruses: Largest viruses Envelope$^+$ with double-stranded DNA; linear, DNA-dependent RNA polymerase in cytoplasm. Transmitted via respiratory droplets or skin lesions, oropharynx epithelium → local lymph nodes → liver and spleen skin → macular, papular, vesicular rash with pustules, crusting

Diagnosis: Increase in titre of antibody, microscopy, looks like herpes but not vesicular

Treatment: None; vaccine used to eradicate; Edward Jenner observed that milkmaids never contracted smallpox virus; secondary to cowpox infection, which acted as a vaccine with antibody cross-reactivity

JC virus

Disease: Progressive multifocal leukoencephalopathy (PML) by demyelination of white matter in AIDS, immunocompromised patients; opportunistic virus, 75% of sera have Ab to JC virus

Prions

Disease: Kuru; progressive tremors, ataxia, no dementia
- Fore tribes in **New Guinea** only
- Via **prions** in eating brains

Disease: Creutzfield-Jakob; presenile dementia and ataxia
- **Spongiform** brain
- Worldwide but rare
- Via prions in iatrogenic transplants, operations
- Linked to BSE (mad cow disease)

PARASITES

CHAPTER 19: OPPORTUNISTIC MYCOSES

History of present illness: 34 yo man from Mississippi presents with
fever, cough, hemoptysis, and chest pain for 1 week. He has no history
of asthma, but has an inspiratory stridor and wheezing characteristic
of allergic bronchopulmonary disease. Sinusitis with localized pain is
also present. CXR shows a lesion in the upper left lobe (Figure 19.1).

Aspergillus fumigatus (Figure 19.2)
Disease: Aspergillosis
Characteristics and pathogenesis: Mold only; not dimorphic, with
septate hyphae in V-shaped branches, conidia form radiating
chains; transmitted as airborne conidia → colonize abraded skin,
wounds, burns → disseminate and form **fungal ball** lesions (lung
granulomas) (Figure 19.3).
Diagnosis: blue-green colonies on culture; septate hyphae

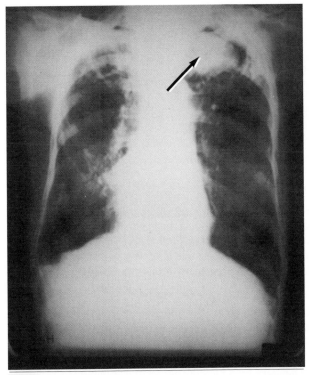

FIGURE 19.1 Fungal ball lesions of *Aspergillosis.*

PARASITES

OPPORTUNISTIC MYCOSES—cont'd

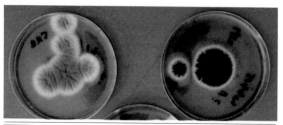

FIGURE 19.2   *Aspergillus* in culture.

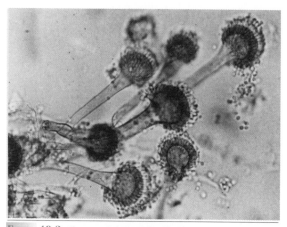

FIGURE 19.3   Characteristic conidia of *Aspergillus*.

History of present illness: 42 yo AIDS patient presents with white oral mucosal patches of 1 week duration. In addition, the patient has had retrosternal pain and difficulty swallowing. Fever and chills without nausea and vomiting are present and have been unresponsive to antibiotic therapy. Her problems are further exacerbated by a vulvo-vaginal pruritis, edema, and erythema with white discharge.

Candida albicans (Figure 19.4)
Disease: Candidiasis; oropharyngeal thrush (Figure 19.5), esophagitis, vulvovaginitis, disseminated candidiasis
Characteristics and pathogenesis: Budding yeast and **pseudohyphae** with **chlamydaspore** formation (Figure 19.6) transmitted by health care workers; part of endogenous flora of immunocompromised and diabetic patients
Diagnosis: Clinical, cultures
Treatment: clotrimazole, nystatin, ketoconazole

OPPORTUNISTIC MYCOSES—cont'd

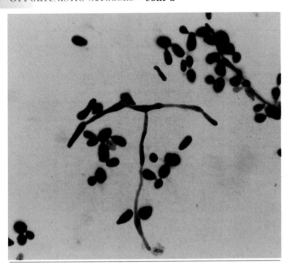

FIGURE 19.4   *Candida albicans.*

PARASITES

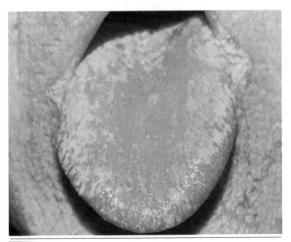

FIGURE 19.5   Oropharyngeal thrush.

OPPORTUNISTIC MYCOSES—cont'd

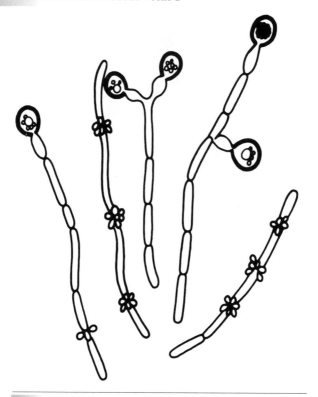

FIGURE 19.6 Pseudohyphae with chlamydaspore formation.

History of present illness: 42 yo AIDS patient who states he was
smelling "pidgeon poop," presents with fever to 39° C, nuchal rigidity,
headache, and general malaise. He has been unable to think clearly
and states that his vision is going. He has been noncompliant with his
medication. A rash resembling molluscum contagiosum has erupted
on his face (Figure 19.7). Spinal tap is negative for bacteria.

Cryptococcus neoformans
Disease: Cryptococcosis: meningitis
Characteristics and pathogenesis: Oval budding yeast with a polysaccharide capsule, found in soil contaminated with **pigeon
droppings** → inhalation and dissemination of conidia → pneumonia,
meningitis, especially in immunocompromised
Diagnosis: Latex agglutination detection of capsular antigen in CSF,
stained with **India ink** (Figure 19.8); **grown in thistle seed medium**
Treatment: fluconazole

OPPORTUNISTIC MYCOSES—cont'd

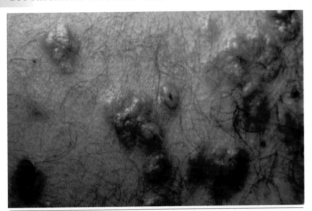

FIGURE 19.7 Dermatologic manifestation of cryptococcal infection.

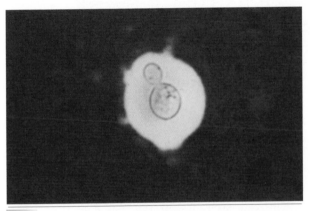

FIGURE 19.8 India ink stain of *Cryptococcus.*

PARASITES

OPPORTUNISTIC MYCOSES—cont'd

History of present illness: 46 yo diabetic patient presents with a
"**black nose.**" The patient's symptoms began with sinusitis. After 3
days, the infection spread, causing necrosis and lack of circulation in
the nasal and periocular vasculature. Fever and a large **telangiecta-
sia** of the roof of the mouth are noted (Figure 19.9).

Rhizopus, Mucor, or ***Absidia*** fungi
Disease: Mucormycosis or zygomycosis
Characteristics and pathogenesis: Inhaled fungi proliferate in blood
    vessels → cause **necrosis** and infection → **rhinocerebral** mucormy-
    cosis (most common) in diabetics, **90-degree** nonseptate hyphae,
    enclosed in a sporangium
Diagnosis: Clinical and biopsy specimens
Treatment: Surgical resection; amphotecin B at diagnosis; hyperbaric
    oxygen in some cases

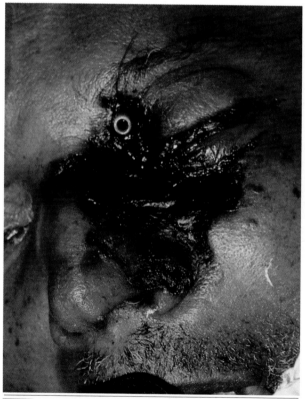

FIGURE 19.9 "Black nose" of mucormycosis.

CHAPTER 20: SUPERFICIAL MYCOSES

History of present illness: 5 yo presents with an itchy and flaky rash on the occipital region of the head. In addition, there is a patch of baldness in the circumscribed regions. On the extremities, a reddish, ring-like rash that has a burning sensation is noted. The regions are dry and pruritic.

Dermatophytoses: *Microsporum, Trichophyton, Epidermophyton*
(Figure 20.1)
Tinea capitis: scalp (Figure 20.2)
Tinea cruris: jock itch (Figure 20.3)
Tinea pedis: athlete's foot (Figure 20.4)
Tinea unguim: nails (Figure 20.5)
Disease: Ringworm; jock itch; athlete's foot
Characteristics and pathogenesis: Organism infects superficial keratinized structures by direct contact; flourish in moist environments
Diagnosis: 10% KOH, **wood's light, Sabouraud's** agar
Treatment: Miconazole, ketoconozale, griseofulvin (when severe)

PARASITES

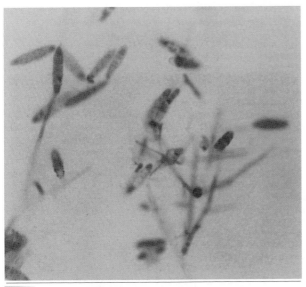

FIGURE 20.1 *Microsporum.*

SUPERFICIAL MYCOSES—cont'd

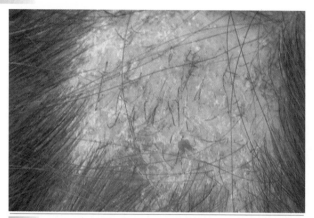

FIGURE 20.2   Tinea capitis.

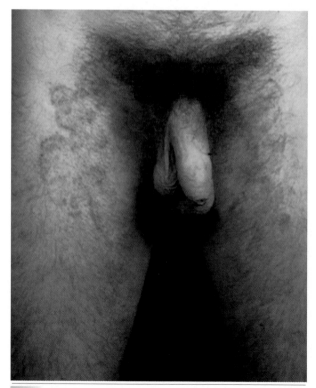

FIGURE 20.3   Tinea cruris.

SUPERFICIAL MYCOSES—cont'd

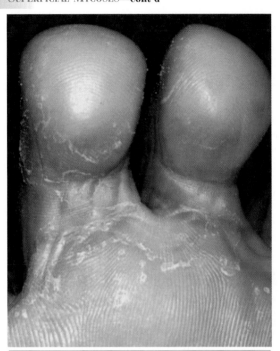

FIGURE 20.4   Tinea pedis.

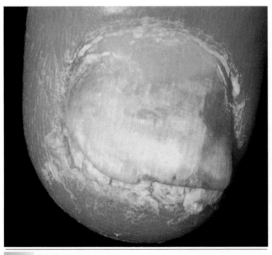

FIGURE 20.5   Tinea unguim.

PARASITES

History of present illness: 24 yo **gardener** presents with a small red painless bump resembling an insect bite on the third finger of the right upper extremity. He stubbed that finger on a **rose thorn** 5 weeks earlier. The bump has opened and new nodules have appeared. There are boils with many regions of ulceration along that extremity (Figure 20.6).

Sporothrix schenckii
Disease: Sporotrichosis
Characteristics and pathogenesis: Round cigar-shaped budding yeast (Figure 20.7)
Diagnosis: Fungal culture of ulcerated lesion
Treatment: Potassium iodide, itraconazole

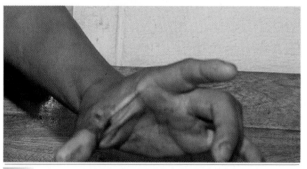

Figure 20.6 *Sporothrix* lesion. © *Dr. Roger Smalligan.*

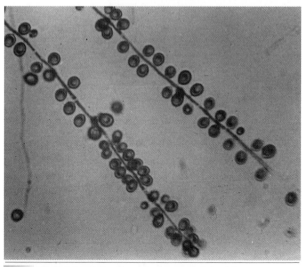

Figure 20.7 Sporothrix schenckii: characteristic budding morphology.

CHAPTER 21: SYSTEMIC MYCOSES

History of present illness: 44 yo forestry worker from **Ohio and Mississippi river valleys** presents with dry cough with no sputum production and mild fever to 39° C of 3 weeks duration. He has had occasional dysuria and mild arthralgias. A small skin rash is noted on the lower right side of the face (Figure 21.1).

Blastomyces dermatidis

Disease: Blastomycosis: pulmonary, skin, bone, GU infections

Characteristics and pathogenesis: Dimorphic fungus, mold in soil, yeast in tissue, telomeric growth with a round refractive wall out of which a single **broad-based bud** forms (Figure 21.2). Transmitted via inhalation of **conidia** → asymptomatic unless immunocompromised → dissemination to form skin and bone granulomas, genitourinary infections

Diagnosis: Complement fixation and immunodiffusion

Treatment: ketoconazole

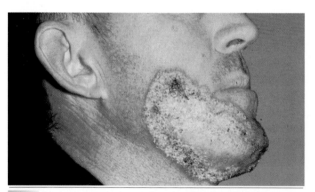

FIGURE 21.1 Dermatologic manifestations of blastomycosis.

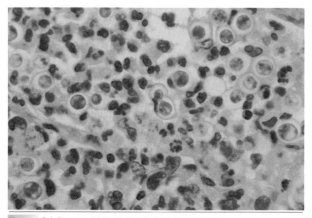

FIGURE 21.2 Broad-based budding of *Blastomyces.*

PARASITES

SYSTEMIC MYCOSES—cont'd

History of present illness: 35 yo **AIDS** patient from **Arizona** presents with influenza-like illness with fever, cough, headaches, rash, and myalgias of 2 weeks duration. Chest auscultation reveals bronchi in the left lobes, verified by CXR as a pneumonia. In addition, the patient complains of **arthralgias** of the upper and lower extremity joints and red nodules **(erythema nodosum)** on the wrists.

Coccidioides immitis
Disease: Coccidiomycosis; valley fever
Characteristics and pathogenesis: Dimorphic fungus that lives as a mold in soil and spherule in tissue; transmitted from soil → inhaled → spherules form and rupture → disseminate to bone, CNS, lungs (Figure 21.3)
Diagnosis: Skins tests: **coccidioidin** and **spherulin** (growth filtrates); Ab tests: tube precipitation; complement fixation
Treatment: amphotericin B, ketoconazole, fluconazole (with meningitis)

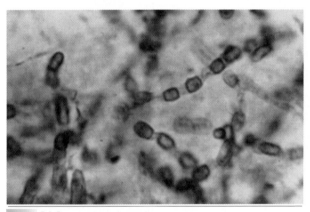

FIGURE 21.3 *Coccidiodes immitis.*

SYSTEMIC MYCOSES—cont'd

History of present illness: 39 yo cleaner of bat and bird droppings develops fever, chest pains, and dry or nonproductive cough. The patient does not respond to antibiotic treatment. A zealous pulmonologist takes a biospy, which when cultured reveals the following organism:

Histoplasma capsulatum
Disease: Histoplasmosis (Figure 21.4)
Characteristics and pathogenesis: Dimorphic fungus: mold in soil → yeast in tissue, transmitted as microconidia → inhaled → enter macrophages → become yeast → 95% of patients asymptomatic from encased granulomas with calcification → dissemination otherwise in immunocompromised patients
Diagnosis: Oval budding yeasts within macrophages
Positive complement fixation test, positive **histoplasmin** skin test
Treatment: ketoconazole, amphotericin B (when severe)

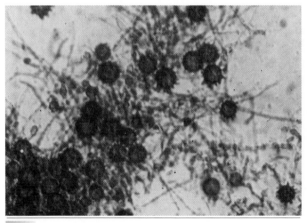

FIGURE 21.4 *Histoplasma capsulatum.*

PARASITES

CHAPTER 22: CESTODES (TAPEWORMS)

History of present illness: 42 yo man in Ecuador, working as a dog and sheep breeder, presents with fever to 39° C of 1 week duration, with abdominal and right upper quadrant pain, and a positive Murphy's sign. He has also had chest pain, cough, and hemoptysis for 1 week. Ultrasound examination confirms a mass in the hepatic area and biliary duct obstruction.

Echinococcus granulosus (dog tapeworm)

Disease: Echinococcosis, hydatid cyst disease (Figures 22.1 and 22.2)

Characteristics and pathogenesis: Cycles among sheep and dogs, but if eggs are accidentally eaten by humans, **hydatid cysts** form in liver, brain, lungs, bone, and heart. Rupture of cysts produces fever, urticaria, eosinophilia, and anaphylactic shock, and cyst dissemination.

Diagnosis: Ultrasound; aspiration of liver cyst: "**Hydatid sand**"; Fluid aspirated from a hydatid cyst will show multiple **protoscolices with hooklets**

Treatment: previously only surgery, but now benzimidazole therapy and puncture (of cysts), aspiration, injection, and re-aspiration **(PAIR)** procedures

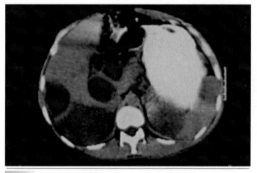

FIGURE 22.1 Hydatid cyst disease.

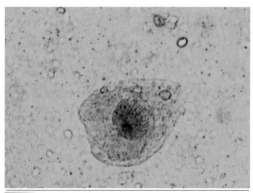

FIGURE 22.2 *Echinococcus.*

CESTODES (TAPEWORMS)—cont'd

History of present illness: 42 yo man in Ecuador presents with abdominal pain of 2 days duration. He has had no fever, chills, vomiting, and only minor diarrhea. Symptoms began after the ingestion of raw beef at the Quichua harvest festival. PE is unremarkable.

Taenia saginata (beef tapeworm) (Figure 22.3)
Disease: Taeniasis; no cysticercosis
Characteristics and pathogenesis: Scolex has four muscular suckers with no hooklets; eggs eaten by cattle → larvae (cysticerus) in beef → **raw beef** eaten by humans → adults worm in human intestine → minor symptoms
Diagnosis: Stool microscopy, **gravid proglottids** (central stem with numerous lateral branches) observed; antibody detection
Treatment: praziquantel

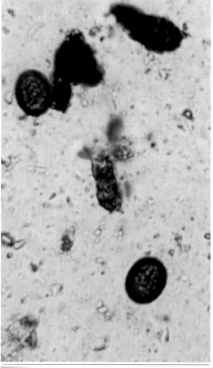

FIGURE 22.3 *Taenia saginata* eggs.

History of present illness: 42 yo man in Ecuador presents with abdominal pain of 2 days duration. He has had fever, chills, vomiting, headache, and loss of consciousness. Friends state that he has been seizing with losses of consciousness for the past 8 hours. Patient also complains of blurry vision. All symptoms began after consumption of cuy; a local pork delicacy. PE reveals mild nuchal rigidity. A CT shows multiple calcified cystic lesions (Figure 22.4).

Taenia solium (pork tapeworm)

Disease: Cysticercosis (larvae infection); CNS involvement includes parenchymal cysts → seizures, meningitis, hydrocephalus, retinitis or **taeniasis (adult** infection)

Characteristics and pathogenesis: Scolex with four suckers and circle of **hooks; eggs** eaten by humans → disseminate to eyes and brain → encystations as cysticeri → calcified brain lesions → symptoms

Diagnosis: Stool microscopy, gravid proglottids observed with few lateral branches; clinical diagnosis with CT

Treatment: praziquantel

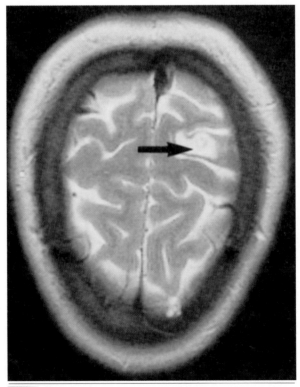

FIGURE 22.4 Cysticerosis lesion of the brain. © *Dr. Roger Smalligan.*

CHAPTER 23: NEMATODES (ROUNDWORMS)—INTESTINAL

History of present illness: 5 yo child presents with severe abdominal
pain for 2 weeks of increasing intensity. Abdominal x-ray shows distended loops of bowel with many air/fluid signs. The patient also presents with right upper quadrant pain. An ultrasound of the region
shows migrating worms obstructing the biliary tract. In addition, the
patient has had pulmonary symptoms (e.g., cough, dyspnea, hemoptysis) for many weeks. One worm is recovered from the appendix of the
patient (Figure 23.1).

Ascaris lumbricoides (Figure 23.2)
Disease: Ascariasis; secondary bowel and **biliary tract** obstruction,
   eosinophilic pneumonitis (**Loeffler's** syndrome).
Characteristics and pathogenesis: Fecal/oral transmission → eggs
   ingested → larvae hatch and penetrate GI →bloodstream to lung →
   develop in sputum → swallowed as adult in intestine → eggs in feces
Diagnosis: Wet mount of organism from stool and aspirate; kato-katz
   assessment for quantitation
Treatment: mebendazole or pyrantel pamoate or albendazole

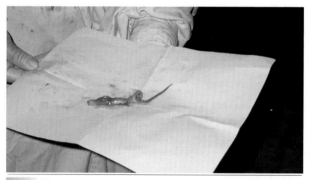

FIGURE 23.1 *Ascaris* worm recovered from surgery. © *Dr. Roger
         Smalligan.*

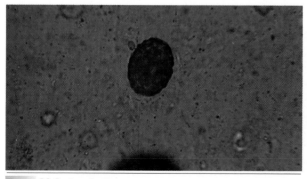

FIGURE 23.2 *Ascaris* egg.

NEMATODES (ROUNDWORMS)—INTESTINAL—cont'd

History of present illness: 35 yo woman presents with a low hematocrit. Her stool has been irregular with diarrhea, although without gross blood. A guiac test is positive, however. In addition, she complains of pruritis of her lower extremities. She has a slight cough, although the lungs appear to be clear upon physical examination. Eosinophilia is present.

Ancylostoma duodenale or *Necator americanus*

Disease: Hookworm infection; secondary iron deficiency anemia via GI blood loss of attachment of worms; GI, cardiac, nutritional, pulmonary, skin manifestations are all possible, secondary to larvae infection

Characteristics and pathogenesis: Larvae penetrate skin, usually at foot, → travel by blood to lungs (**Loeffler's**) → coughed up and eaten as adult→ mate in GI tract, sucking buccal teeth → bleeding and iron deficiency anemia

Diagnosis: Wet mount of stool

Treatment: mebendazole, pyrantel pamoate, or albendazole

◆   ◆   ◆

History of present illness: 6 yo child complains of perianal pruritus for 2 weeks. His mother states, "He picks his butt a lot more at night." Physical exam reveals numerous excoriations. the patient appears irritable with slight abdominal tenderness.

Enterobius vermicularis (pinworm) (Figure 23.3)

Disease: Enterobiasis (pinworm infection)

Characteristics and pathogenesis: Fecal and oral transmission; eggs in environment → eaten, eggs hatch in GI tract → adult → gravid female worm goes to anus → deposits eggs → **itchy butt,** found in > 35% of U.S. school children

Diagnosis: Cellulose tape swab ("Scotch tape test")

Treatment: pyrantel pamoate, mebendazole, or albendazole

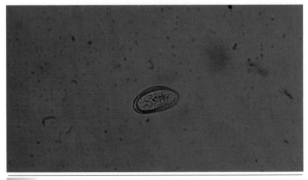

FIGURE 23.3 *Enterobius* egg.

NEMATODES (ROUNDWORMS)—INTESTINAL—cont'd

History of present illness: 42 yo man from rural Arkansas presents with gastrointestinal symptoms that include abdominal pain and diarrhea. In addition, a dry cough without any sputum production is noted. Dermatologic symptoms include urticarial rashes in the buttocks and waist areas, which have not resolved with hydrocortisone. Blood work shows hypereosinophilia.

Strongyloides stercoralis (Figure 23.4): Found in tropics, Southeast Asia, southern United States; wherever feces is used as fertilizer

Disease: Strongyloidiasis; **Loffler's syndrome:** pneumonitis; eosinophilia. In immunocompromised patients: disseminated strongyloidiasis → liver, heart, kidney, CNS

Characteristics and pathogenesis: two life cycles; live in humans (female lays eggs); in soil as male and female → mate → larvae penetrate unbroken skin via soil → carried to lung → swallowed larvae → into intestine as adult → back to lung as larvae

Diagnosis: identification of larvae via duodenal fluid **String test; Baermann** funnel technique; **Harada-Mori** filter paper technique

Treatment: ivermectin, thiabendazole, and albendazole

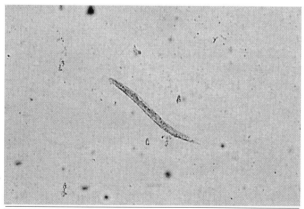

FIGURE 23.4 *Strongyloides stercoralis.*

CHAPTER 24: NEMATODES—TISSUE

History of present illness: 45 yo farm worker traveling between **Yemen** and **Togo** complains of a painful ulcer of 2 weeks duration on the right foot. A whitish worm emerged in the center of the lesion, which was subsequently followed by swelling and inflammation. The area is tender to touch, and patient is mildly febrile.

Dracunculiasis medinemsis
Disease: Dracunculiasis (guinea fire worm disease)
Characteristics and pathogenesis: Transmitted as **copepod** (in unfiltered water) consumed; develop to larvae stage; nodules **poke out as worm creates ulcer**
Diagnosis: Head of worm in ulcer (eeyuww!)
Treatment: Pull out on stick for 2 to 4 cm per day

♦   ♦   ♦

History of present illness: 18 yo man from Botswana complains of something moving in his eye. Further examination reveals **subconjunctival movement** of a **worm**. No other symptoms are present and the patient is healthy otherwise. Eosinophilia is noted on blood work.

Loa loa
Disease: Loiasis in Central and West Africa; episodic angioedema (**Calabar** swellings) and subconjunctival migration
Characteristics and pathogenesis: Deer fly (mango fly) vector → deposit larvae on skin → enter wound → adults → females produce microfilia during **day (sheathed)** → migrate in subcutaneous tissue over nose through eye → itching → Calabar swellings
Diagnosis: Blood smear for microfilia
Treatment: diethylcarbamazine

NEMATODES—TISSUE—cont'd

History of present illness: 14 yo adolescent who was swimming in the Congo River presents with pruritus, dermatitis, subcutaneous nodules, and lymphadenopathies of the upper extremities of 4 weeks duration. During this time, her sight has been deteriorating. Eosinophilia is noted with blood analysis.

Oncocerca volvulus

Disease: River blindness; onchocerciasis (Figure 24.1)

Characteristics and pathogenesis: Black fly vector that harbors around rivers in Africa and Central America → bites and transmits vector → adult worms lives in **subcutaneous** tissue → **nonsheathed microfilaria** die → concentrated in eye → lesions of cornea, iris → total blindness, pruritis, pigmentation, edema, → onchocercal dermatitis/hanging groin

Diagnosis: Tissue excision, skin biopsies, and microscopy of microfilaria

Treatment: ivermectin, not diethylcarbamizine; kills microfilaria (worse symptoms)

PARASITES

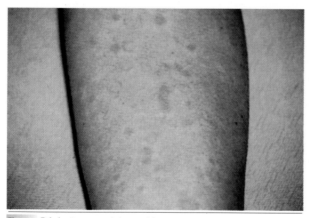

FIGURE 24.1 Oncocercal dermatitis.

NEMATODES—TISSUE—cont'd

History of present illness: 5 yo boy presents with fever, anorexia, weight loss, cough, wheezing, and other generalized asthmatic symptoms. Physical exam reveals an abdominal normal reticular rash and hepatosplenomegaly. The left foot appears to be severely infected. There is extreme pruritis. Blood count reveals hypereosinophilia.

Toxocera canis
Disease: Two forms
(1) **Ocular larva migrans** (OLM): Retinal inflammation by worm → blindness
(2) **Visceral larva migrans** (VLM): Heavy *Toxocara* infection → worm burden → **inflammation** of organs as worm **moves** through body
Characteristics and pathogenesis: fecal oral transmission from dog host → GI → then liver, brain, eyes
Diagnosis: larvae in biopsied tissue, **hypergammaglobulinemia,** eosinophilia
Treatment: diethylcarbamazine

◆   ◆   ◆

History of present illness: 32 yo man in rural Thailand complains of swelling of the legs and scrotum. Physical exam reveals tender lymph nodes to palpation and severe edema in both lower extremities and **scrotum.** In addition, patient is febrile (38.7° C) and uncomfortable. Blood work shows an elevated eosinophil count.

Wucheria bancrofti (also *Brugia malayi*)
Disease: Lymphatic filariasis: **chyluria, elephantiasis,** edema
Characteristics and pathogenesis: Female *Anopheles* mosquito drops larvae on skin while biting → lymph nodes → mature adults making microfilaria → microfilaria die to cause pathology → edema, lymphadenitis, hydrocele, chyluria, elephantiasis
Diagnosis: Because of **nocturnal** activity of organism, must know periodicity when taking blood for smear or use diethylcarbamazine for provocative challenge and bait to periphery → concentrate blood via centrifugation of sample lysed in 2% formalin (**Knott's** technique), PCR/antigen detection
Treatment: diethylcarbamazine or ivermectin

CHAPTER 25: TREMATODES (FLUKES)

History of present illness: 42 yo man in Kyoto, Japan, presents with abdominal pain, nausea, diarrhea of 1 week duration, after having eaten bad sushi. RUQ pain has become more severe, and he has a positive Murphy's sign. Eosinophilia is noted with the CBC.

Clonorchis sinesis

Disease: Chlonorchiasis (Oriental liver fluke) infection, secondary cholangitis, cholelithiasis, pancreatitis, and cholangiocarcinoma

Characteristics and pathogenesis: Undercooked fish → larvae excyst in duodenum → immature **flukes** enter biliary ducts → obstruct biliary tract **(cholangitis)** adults make eggs → leave as feces into fresh water snails → eggs hatch into larvae → feces swimming **cercariae** → underscales of fish → cycle again

Diagnosis: Eggs in stool or duodenal aspirate

Treatment: praziquantel or albendazole

◆   ◆   ◆

History of present illness: 45 yo man in Bangalore, India, presents with diarrhea, abdominal pain, fever to 39° C, and cough with hemoptysis after having eaten raw crabs. Urticaria and hepatosplenomegaly are also found on PE. Mild rales are noted bilaterally; eosinophilia is observed in the blood differential. (The CXR is shown in Figure 25.1.)

Paragonimus westermani (lung fluke)

Disease: Paragonimiasis

Characteristics and pathogenesis: Prevalent in Asia and India; undercooked **crabmeat** → larvae that excyst in small intestine → loose penetration into GI wall → migrate **through diaphragm** into lung → eggs coughed up, swallowed, and excreted

Diagnosis: Operculated eggs in sputum or feces

Treatment: praziquantel, bithionol

PARASITES

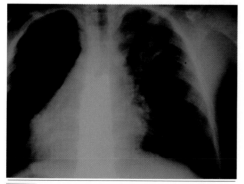

FIGURE 25.1 CXR of paragonimiasis. © Dr. Roger Smalligan.

TREMATODES (FLUKES)—cont'd

History of present illness: 28 yo man presents with a 2 cm lesion on the left lower extremity. In addition, patient has had fever, cough, abdominal pain, and diarrhea with blood for 3 weeks. Patient has complained of forgetfulness and occasional disorientation. PE reveals hepatosplenomegaly and blood work shows eosinophilia.

Schistosoma mansoni, S. japonicum, S. haematobium (Figure 25.2)

Disease: Schistosomiasis; cercarial dermatitis; acute schistosomiasis (**Katayama's** fever) by *S. mansoni* and *S. japonicum;* other secondary disease: colonic polyposis with bloody diarrhea *(S. mansoni);* portal hypertension *(S. mansoni, S. japonicum);* **cystitis** and **ureteritis** *(S. haematobium)* → bladder cancer; pulmonary hypertension *(S. mansoni, S. japonicum);* glomerulonephritis; and CNS lesions

Characteristics and pathogenesis: Penetration of skin by free swimming **cercariae** → larvae → vasculature → mate in portal veins → eggs in vasculature → dissemination to liver, spleen → granulomas → fibrosis → hepatosplenomegaly via portal hypertension

Diagnosis: Eggs in feces or urine *(S. haematobium)* can quantify with Kato-Katz or Ritchie technique

Treatment: praziquantel

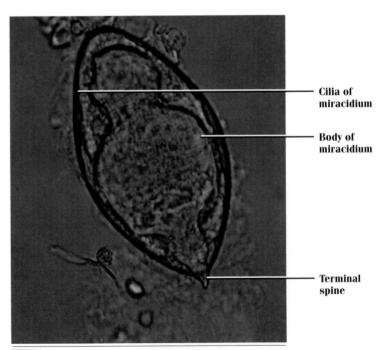

Cilia of miracidium

Body of miracidium

Terminal spine

FIGURE 25.2 *Schistosoma mansoni.*

CHAPTER 26: PROTOZOA—BLOOD AND TISSUE

History of present illness: 42 yo South American woman complains of mouth lesions of 1 month duration. Her appetite is significantly decreased with a mild intermittent fever. Her neighbors state that she has lost a lot of weight and appears darker in complexion. PE reveals hepatosplenomegaly and numerous punctate lesions in the mucosal membranes in the oropharynx. The right side of the face and ear have many ulcerated lesions (Figure 26.1).

Leishmania donovani (Figure 26.2)

Disease: Visceral leishmaniasis **(kala-azar "black fever"):** skin hyperpigmentation and fever, RES (reticuloendothelial system) organs affected → liver, spleen, bone marrow → anemia, leukopenia, thrombocytopenia → bleeding, splenomegaly

Characteristics and pathogenesis: Life cycle: female **sandfly** ingests macrophages containing **amastigotes** (no flagellae) → promastigotes (flagellated) in gut → multiply in mouth → bite transmission to human. Enter macrophages via **gp63 (glycoprotein) and LPG** (live as amastigotes in human macrophages)

Diagnosis: Giemsa stained smears of tissue scrapings or aspirates; biopsy material for amastigotes; Leishman-Donovan bodies

Treatment: sodium stibogluconate or meglumine antimonate

PARASITES

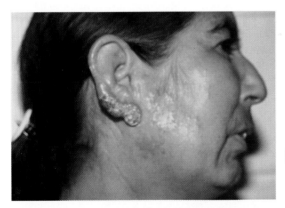

FIGURE 26.1
Clinical presentation of leichmaniasis.
© *Dr. Roger Smalligan.*

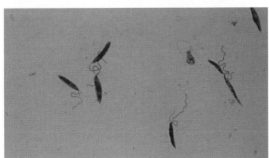

FIGURE 26.2
Leishmania donovani.

History of present illness: 45 yo patient presents in the Amazon jungle hospital with fever and chills of 1 week duration, accompanied by headache, myalgias, arthralgias, weakness, vomiting, and diarrhea (without blood). Other clinical features noted on PE include splenomegaly and tender abdomen. Blood work shows anemia, thrombocytopenia, hypoglycemia, and elevated BUN/creatinine levels.

Plasmodium: *P. vivax, P. ovale, P. malaria, P. falciparum* (most severe malaria, infects all stages of RBC development) (Figures 26.3–26.5)

Disease: Malaria, most common lethal disease (200 million) in the world; clinical presentation can vary substantially depending on the infecting species, *P. falciparum:* fatal; CNS involvement (cerebral malaria), acute renal failure, severe anemia, or adult respiratory distress syndrome; *P. vivax:* **splenomegaly** (splenic rupture, rare) *P. malaria:* **nephrotic** syndrome

Characteristics and pathogenesis: Transmitted human to human via female anopheles mosquito. Two-phase life cycle: **schizogony** (asexual in humans) and **sporogony** sexual in mosquitoes → merozoites into M+F gametocytes in RBC → taken up by mosquitos → fertilization in gut → haploid sporozoites made → salivary glands → bite humans → **exoerythrocytic** phase (sporozoites enter hepatocytes, duplicate into merozoites) → **erythrocytic** phase (merozoites invade RBCs → differentiate into ring shaped **trophozoite** → differentiate into schizont with multiple merozoites) → rupture of RBCs with release of merozoite → immune response by host → and cycle repeats itself; repetition is what causes the pattern of recurrent **chills** → **fever** → drenching **sweat** → **chills** again

PROTOZOA—BLOOD AND TISSUE—cont'd

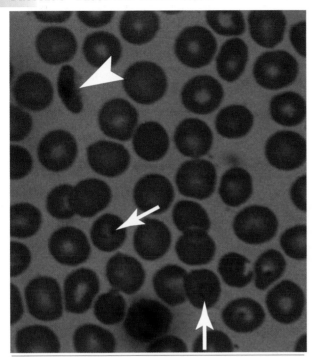

FIGURE 26.3 Trophozoites of *Plasmodium falciparum (arrows)* and a gametoctye *(arrowhead).*

Recurrence:
   (1) Recrudescence: controllable number of parasites in bloodstream → latent in RBC (erythrocytic)
   (2) Relapse: sporozoites dormant in liver → reactivate from **hypnozoites** (exoerythrocytic)
Malarial **resistance in sickle cell patients** since insufficient ATP produced in RBCs to support parasite growth
Diagnosis: Thick and thin smears with Giemsa stain, malarial pigment (hemozoin) in RBC degraded cells; diamond ring-shaped trophozoites within RBCs
Treatment: chloroquine kills sporozoites, sulfadoxine-pyrimethamine, quinine, tetracycline, doxycycline, mefloquine, and primaquine

PARASITES

PROTOZOA—BLOOD AND TISSUE—cont'd

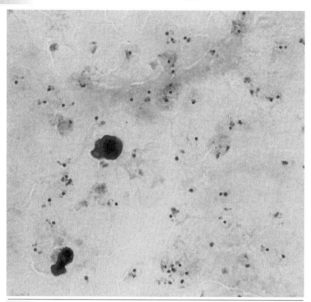

FIGURE 26.4 *Plasmodium vivax* in red blood cells.

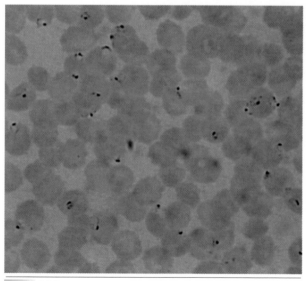

FIGURE 26.5 Schizont differentiation.

PROTOZOA—BLOOD AND TISSUE—cont'd

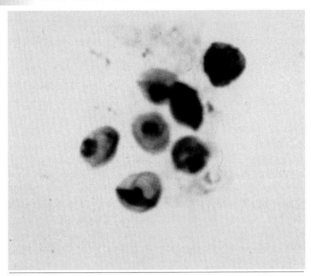

FIGURE 26.6 High magnification.

PARASITES

History of present illness: 32 yo AIDS patient presents with dyspnea, nonproductive cough, and fever to 39° C. CXR demonstrates bilateral infiltrates in all lobes. Sputum and bacterial specimens are negative for TB.

Pneumocystis carinii (Figure 26.6)
Disease: PCP, pneumonia in AIDS
Characteristics and pathogenesis: Classified as **fungus** by rRNA, normally part of endogenous flora, transmission by respiratory inhalation → cysts of sporozoites, in alveoli → exudative inflammation → frothy mucus
Diagnosis: Clinical diagnosis or sputum or bronchoalveolar lavage shows cysts by **silver stain;** Giemsa stain
Treatment: trimethoprim-sulfamethoxazole, pentamidine, atovaquone

PROTOZOA—BLOOD AND TISSUE—cont'd

History of present illness: 45 yo AIDS patient playing with **cats**, and eating **uncooked meat** presents with cervical lymphadenopathy and an influenza-like illness for the last 3 weeks. The patient complains of not being able to think clearly, loss of motor function in the right upper extremity, and general malaise. On PE, patient is tachycardic and rales are heard bilaterally in various lung quadrants. Head CT scan shows a well-circumscribed lesion in the left parietal lobe.

Toxoplasma gondii → infects any nucleated cell
Disease: Toxoplasmosis → toxoplasmic **encephalitis,** myocarditis, pneumonitis, brain lesions, chorioretinitis, hepatitis, lymphadentis
Characteristics and pathogenesis: Transmitted fecal and orally by domestic cats (definite hosts) → humans intermediate hosts, infected by cysts in undercooked meat or pork, contact with cat feces → invade gut mucosa, ingested by macrophages → differentiate to **tachyzoites;** invade brain and muscle → asymptomatic or heterophil negative mononucleosis; life threatening encephalitis in immunocompromised patients because of reactivation of dormant cysts **(bradyzoites)**; transplacental transmission from mother, only if infected in pregnancy → fetal infections → abortion, neonatal encephalitis
Diagnosis: ⇑ IgM; crescent-shaped trophozoites (tachyzoites)
Treatment: Healthy patients need no treatment, otherwise spiramycin or pyrimethamine plus sulfadiazine

♦   ♦   ♦

History of present illness: 32 yo man from East Africa develops a chancre on the left lower extremity of 2 weeks duration. Subsequently, symptoms that include fever, lymphadenopathy, pruritus began in this region. In addition, the patient complained of headaches and somnolence and now appears to be in a coma.

Trypanosomiasis ganbiense (humans, **West** Africa)
T. brucei (cattle)
T. rhodesiense (animals, **East** Africa, fatal)
Disease: Sleeping sickness: chancre → hemolymphatic stage → meningoencephalitic stage
Characteristics and pathogenesis: Transmitted by **tsetse** fly → eat trypomastigotes (nondividing stage) → bite, inflammation at site (chancre) → dissemination in blood → (lymph nodes) antigenic variation via **variant surface glycoprotein** (VSG) active rearrangement → cyclical fever → myocarditis and CNS involvement→ lethargy, sleeping, insomnia → somnolence → coma from encephalitis
Diagnosis: Trypomastigotes in blood smear
Treatment: suramin (early treatment only) does not penetrate BBB, therefore not for encephalitis

PROTOZOA—BLOOD AND TISSUE—cont'd

History of present illness: 42 yo woman from Brazil presents with a local lesion and swelling on the left lower extremity and face. She has had fever to 38.8° C and mild anorexia. On PE, lymphadenopathy, mild hepatosplenomegaly, and tachcardia are noted. The patient is treated and released. After 3 years, patient returns with dyspnea, and a cardiomyopathy is diagnosed (Figure 26.7).

T. cruzi

Disease: American trypanosomiasis: **Chagas'** disease (Central and South America)

Characteristics and pathogenesis: Reduviid bug (kissing bug) vector → Eats trypomastigotes → excrete as feces as another meal eaten → into bloodstream at bite site (swelling **chagoma,** periorbital edema)→ **amastigotes** in myocardium and macrophages (RES) → transmission from trypomastigotes into blood again → acute (facial edema, fever, malaise, lymphandenopathy) or chronic (cardiomyopathy, CHF, **mega**syndrome—heart, megaesophagus, megacolon) symptoms

Diagnosis: Five ways
 (1) Fresh anticoagulated blood for motile parasites
 (2) Thin and thick blood smears stained with Giemsa
 (3) **Xenodiagnosis** with clean Reduviid bug
 (4) Isolation of the agent by inoculation into mice
 (5) Culture in specialized media

Treatment: No effective treatment; nifurtimox and benznidazol are best

PARASITES

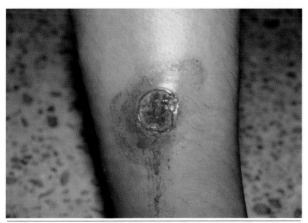

FIGURE 26.7 Characteristic dermatologic presentation of trypanosomiasis.

History of present illness: 32 yo immunocompromised patient presents with watery diarrhea without blood for 2 weeks. Other symptoms include dehydration, weight loss, abdominal pain, fever to 38.8° C, nausea, and vomiting. Patient was self-medicating with Ciprofloxacin to no avail. Other symptoms that began 1 day ago include conjunctival irritation and a slight cough.

Cryptosporidium parvum (Figure 27.1)

Disease: Cryptosporidiosis: watery, **nonbloody** diarrhea, dehydration, malnutrition, lung, **conjunctival** involvement in immunocompromised

Characteristics and pathogenesis: Fecal and oral transmission of oocyst from humans and animals → attached to **jejunum** (no invasion) → **sporozoites** released → intracellular replication in columnar cells →trophozoite → out in stool, persistent in AIDS patients

Diagnosis: Fecal smears → kinyoun acid fast stain or immunofluorescence

Treatment: Supportive measures; sometimes paromomycin

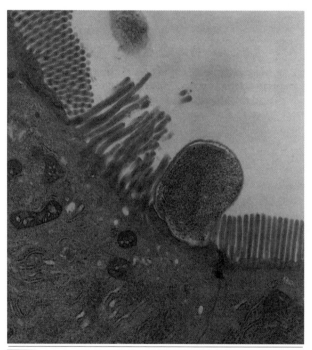

FIGURE 27.1 Cryptosporidium infection of the GI tract.

PARASITES

Protozoa—Intestinal and UG—cont'd

History of present illness: 32 yo traveler in Bangladesh presents with foul smelling diarrhea, abdominal pain, bloating, nausea, and vomiting for 2 weeks. The patient has no blood in the stool, is slightly tachycardic, and has been unable to eat for the last 2 days.

Giardia lamblia (Figure 27.2)

Disease: Giardiasis (nonbloody, greasy, foul-smelling diarrhea with farts, cramps, and more farts)

Characteristics and pathogenesis: Cysts have rigid cell walls, non-dividing; two stages:
  (1) Trophozoite: **pear-shaped,** 2 nuclei, 4 pairs flagellae, **suction disk**
  (2) Cysts: thick-walled oval cyst; 2 nuclei, transmitted as animals pass cyst into water → fecally contaminated food and water → excystation in **duodenum** → flattened villi → inflammation → malabsorption of protein and fat

Diagnosis: String test: trophozoites adhere in stool or ova and parasite tests

Treatment: metronidazole, filter cysts and kill by boiling; no chlorination

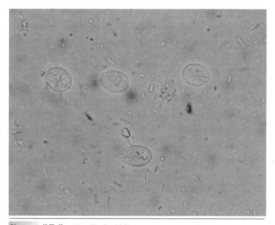

Figure 27.2　*Giardia lamblia.*

PARASITES

PROTOZOA—INTESTINAL AND UG—cont'd

History of present illness: 32 yo traveler develops nausea, loose stools, weight loss, abdominal tenderness and fever to 38.5° C. After 1 week, patient's febrile episodes increase with a temperature elevated to 39.8° C. Patient complains of RUQ pain. On PE, the patient has a positive Murphy's sign, yet an ultrasound shows a completely normal gallbladder.

Entamoeba histolytica (Figure 27.3)
Disease: Amebic dysentery and liver abscess
Characteristics and pathogenesis: Two stages in life cycle
  (1) Motile trophozoite (or amoeba)
  (2) Nonmotile cyst, transmitted fecal/oral via bad food → excystation in ileum → invasion of colon epithelium → necrosis, teardrop ulcer → liver, **no animal** reservoir
Diagnosis: Wet mounts and ova and parasite test; trophozoite has a single nucleus. Ingested RBC cysts are small with **4** nuclei → hatch in GI → **8** trophozoites amebic dysentary has no PMNs in stool, whereas bacterial dysentary does
Treatment: iodoquinol or paromomycin (if asymptomatic); metronidazole or tinidazole (if liver involvement)

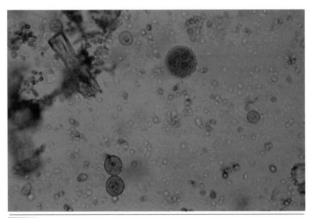

FIGURE 27.3 *Entamoeba histolytica.*

History of present illness: 28 yo woman presents to the OB/GYN clinic with vaginitis for 2 weeks, with a purulent foul-smelling discharge. Other symptoms include dysuria and dyspareunia. PE reveals several vulvar and cervical lesions and abdominal pain with palpation. She is in a monogamous relationship and states that her husband has **no** symptoms.

Trichomonas vaginalis

Disease: Trichomoniasis in women; watery foul-smelling, green vaginal discharge

Heartburn asymptomatic in men, but 10% → urethritis

Characteristics and pathogenesis: Four anterior flagella, undulation membrane → jerky movts, **pear-shaped trophozoite** with central nucleus; no cyst; transmitted by sexual contact → vagina and prostate, predisposition by loss of vaginal acidity

Diagnosis: Wet mount, or for greater sensitivity, direct immunofluorescent antibody culture

Treatment: metronidazole; tinidazole

PARASITES

INDEX